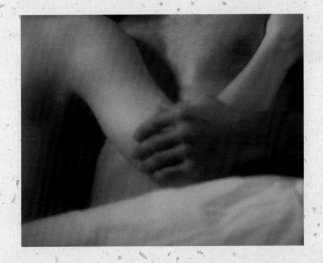

THE *Spirituality* OF SEX

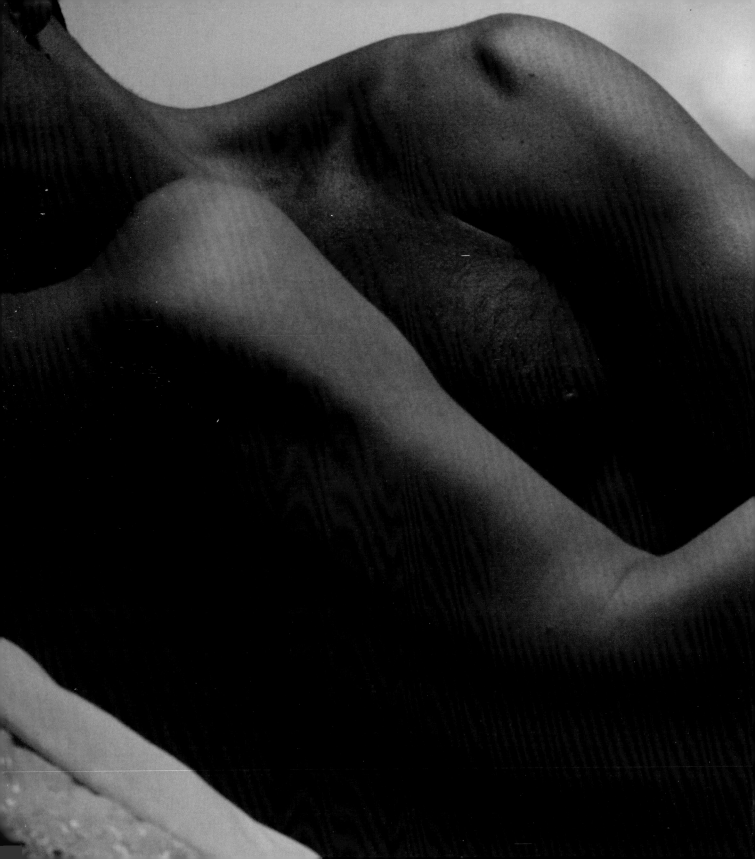

MICHAEL SCHWARTZENTRUBER

MARY MILLERD　　CHARLOTTE JACKSON　　LOIS HUEY-HECK

THE *Spirituality* OF SEX

Northstone

Concept: Northstone Team
Editor: Tim Faller
Cover and Interior design: Verena Velten
Proofreading: Dianne Greenslade
Photo Credits: page 159

Permissions

"Tiny Gods," from the Penguin publication *The Gift: Poems of Hafiz*, copyright 1999 Daniel Ladinsky and used with his permission.

"It Happens All the Time in Heaven," from the Penguin publication *The Subject Tonight Is Love: 60 Wild & Sweet Poems of Hafiz*, copyright 1996 & 2003 Daniel Ladinsky and used with his permission.

"Like This" from the publication *The Essential Rumi*, copyright 1995 Coleman Barks and used with his permission.

NORTHSTONE PUBLISHING is an imprint of WOOD LAKE BOOKS INC. Wood Lake Books acknowledges the financial support of the Government of Canada, through the Book Publishing Industry Development Program (BPIDP) for its publishing activities.

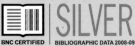

BNC CERTIFIED | SILVER BIBLIOGRAPHIC DATA 2008-09

WOOD LAKE BOOKS INC. is an employee-owned company, committed to caring for the environment and all creation. Wood Lake Books recycles, reuses, and encourages readers to do the same. Resources are printed on recycled paper and more environmentally friendly groundwood papers (newsprint), whenever possible. The trees used are replaced through donations to the Scoutrees For Canada Program. A percentage of all profit is donated to charitable organizations.

Library and Archives Canada Cataloguing in Publication

The spirituality of sex / Michael Schwartzentruber... [et al.].
Includes bibliographical references.
ISBN 978-1-896836-90-4

1. Sex. 2. Spirituality. 3. Sex–Religious aspects. I. Schwartzentruber, Michael, 1960-
BL65.S4S69 2009   306.7   C2009-902762-3

Published by Northstone Publishing
an imprint of WOOD LAKE BOOKS, INC.
9590 Jim Bailey Road, Kelowna, BC, Canada, V4V 1R2
250.766.2778
www.northstone.com
www.woodlakebooks.com

Printing 10 9 8 7 6 5 4 3 2 1
Printed in Canada by Friesens

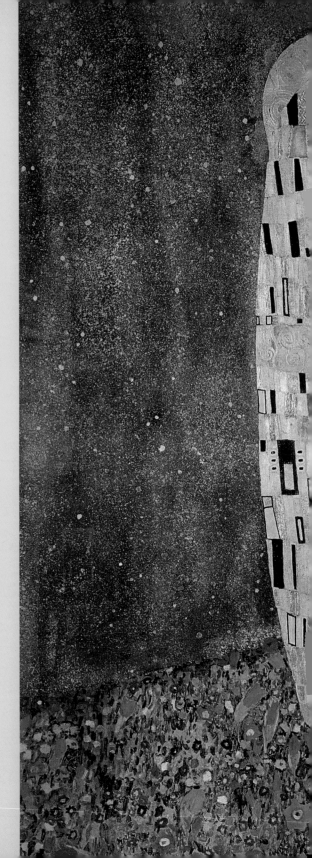

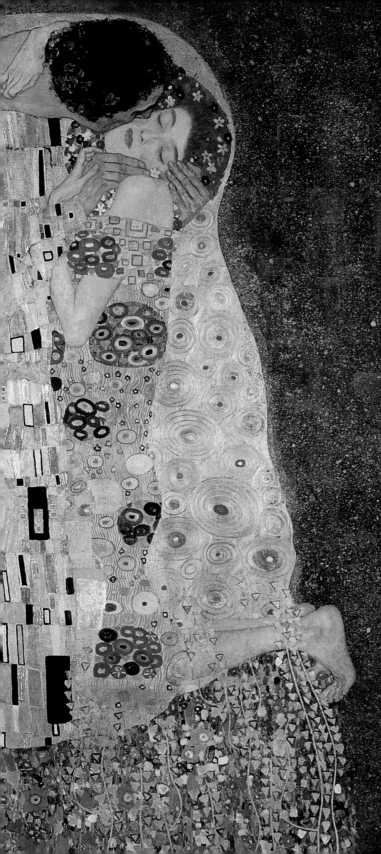

Contents

DEDICATIONS

Michael Schwartzentruber
For Margaret
Spiro and Verena, Anna and Patrick, Jeff and Kathleen

Lois Huey-Heck
For Jim Feather who knows about love
Bryan and Jess
the born and unborn daughters and sons
and to "Lee" one of the lost ones

Charlotte Jackson
For my children, Nellie and Julian

Mary Millerd
To my son, Donnie,
whose death revealed to me the reality and tangibility of spirit

Acknowledgments

MICHAEL SCHWARTZENTRUBER → I want to thank the following people for their role in helping this book come to fruition. Susan Ivany's contribution to this project was much larger than the portions of her writing I have included in Chapter 7, and I am truly grateful. Jim Bell, Tim Scorer, Muriel Bechtel, and Kay Weber reviewed my chapters and offered both encouragement and helpful suggestions, which I have tried to incorporate. Of course, without Lois Huey-Heck, Mary Millerd, and Charlotte Jackson this book would not just be only half as good, it wouldn't exist at all. On behalf of all four of us, I also want to offer our thanks to editor Tim Faller for making our respective manuscripts the best they could be; and to Verena Velten, for making this book the thing of beauty that it is. Finally, I want to thank my wife, Margaret Kyle, who wholeheartedly supported my decision to take on this project. In this, as in the rest of our life together, she brought beauty and inspiration and love.

LOIS HUEY-HECK → Many thanks to readers Merlin Beltain, Grainger Brown, Julie Elliott, Mike Schwartzentruber, and Tim Scorer for caring; Jim for generosity in living with my sophomoric writing-neurosis and the relational feast and famine that accompanied the process; the treasured companions who've helped mend the wounds and make sense of this crazy thing called love; my friends and co-workers at Wood Lake Publishing; and the beloved spiritual companions past, present, and future, including the Pacific Jubilee community, who share the journey.

MARY MILLERD → My appreciation abounds for Tim Scorer who suggested to Mike Schwartzentruber that I write a chapter in the book. Tim's continual encouragement supports me in my work. A big thanks to Mike for asking me and to both Mike and Lois Huey-Heck for their caring support in the writing process. I could not have written this chapter without the love of my family: Don, my husband; and Margot, Jenn, Lisa and Ali. They move my heart and make me feel alive.

CHARLOTTE JACKSON → I would like to acknowledge my teachers: Andrew Feldmar, Father Thomas Keating, Cynthia Bourgeault, and the Ridhwan School; beacons of illumination along the way.

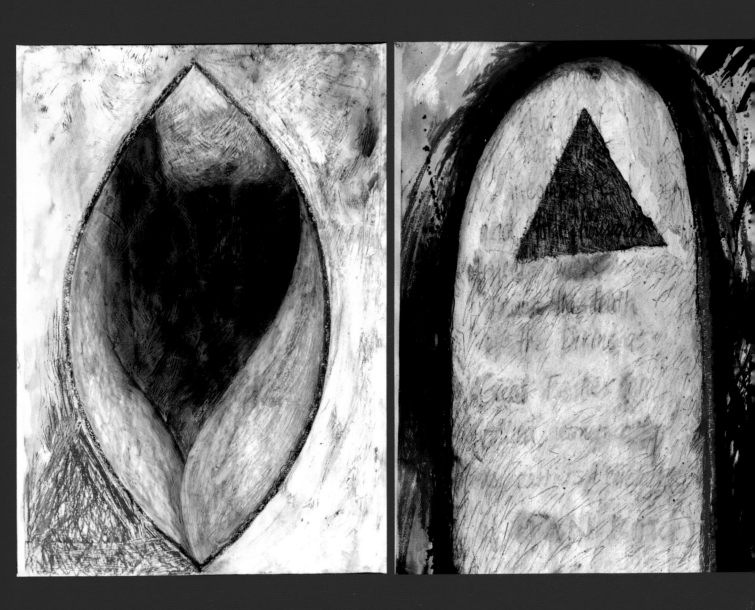

An Invitation into Luscious Wholeness

LOIS HUEY-HECK

Years ago, I started an art piece called "A Ridiculously Abbreviated History of Western Spiritual Understanding." The first image was a symbolic rendering of female genitalia. The caption read something like, "In the beginning, we revered the feminine as Divine and women as creators of life. The role of the male in conception was not understood, and in mythology males were often cast merely as consorts to the Goddess. Our first mistake: we undervalued half of the species."

The second image was a comparable depiction of male genitalia with the caption, "Later, we came to understand that male sperm and semen were required for birth, but decided at the same time that women were merely incubators for the male 'egg.' Men became divinized and God became male. Our second mistake: we devalued the other half of the species."

I imagined that the third image would be a vision of what could be. Not utopia, but a more whole, just, and truthful picture of life. Many times I attempted to capture this "third phase," starting with questions like, "Are we ready now to value female *and* male, matter *and* spirit, body *and* mind?" Despite repeated attempts, I was never satisfied with the images or the text. In retrospect, I realize that I was unable to finish the project because I couldn't say a resounding "yes" to my own questions. Had *I* done the integrative work of bringing together the sexual and spiritual twains (and all their relatives), who we thought would never "meet"? It turns out I still had miles to go in healing the internal split in *me* between spirit and matter. Fortunately, nothing is ever lost or wasted in the economy of Grace.

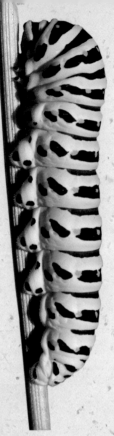
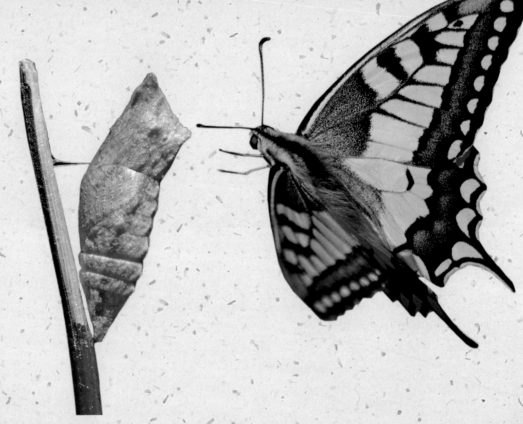

Twenty years – and mountains of spiritual-sexual scholarship, activism, and awakening – later, we are emerging from our earlier caterpillar- and cocoon-like states. It's not always easy work, but the outcome is completely worth the labour.

I revel in knowing that inside a cocoon-of-its-own-making, the caterpillar surrenders its life *so completely* that it dissolves into a fluid state. This is worth repeating: inside its cocoon, a caterpillar surrenders its former life to the extent that it *becomes liquid*. Of its previous eating, drinking, and ambulatory form, all that remains in the chrysalis stage is the essential life force in a formless fluid state. We all know the ever-amazing outcome of the story: how after the wing-strengthening struggle to emerge from the cocoon, the butterfly or moth – our formerly earthbound caterpillar – takes flight. I can't help but notice that while metamorphosis of this magnitude may be free, it doesn't come cheap.

For us mortality-conscious humans, leaving familiar forms requires a profound level of trust. Unlike our caterpillar friends, we're not driven by biological imperative to cocoon, let go, and take flight. Sometimes we begin the transformative process because the old "form" has been too damaging or painful to endure. Sometimes the familiar life has become too small, too confining. At other times, we become aware of an invitation to something bigger than ourselves.

Whatever our impetus for change, most of us need a vision of what's possible before we'll surrender our long-held assumptions and practices. The potential of a nourishing, delicious, and ecstatic spiritual-sexuality can be a big motivator. We believe that the invitation into luscious wholeness is meant for everyone – it is our individual and col-

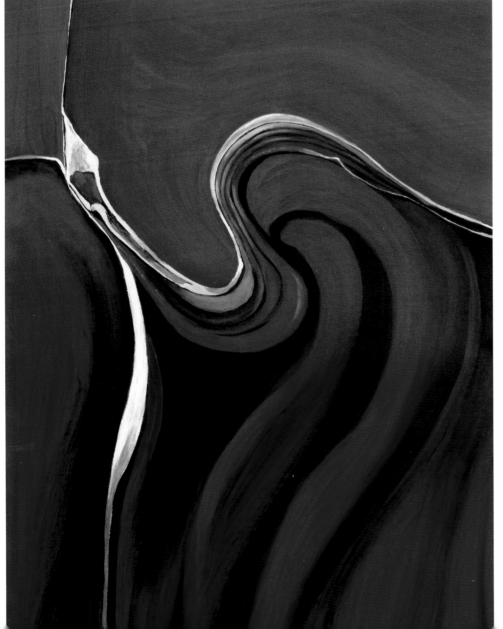

Hope is the celestial and spiritual counterpart of terrestrial and natural instincts of biological reproduction…
In other words, hope is what moves and directs spiritual evolution in the world.

~ Valentin Tomberg

Tomberg calls attention to two aspects of mystical hope. The first is its orientation towards evolution… The world is going somewhere, and that [type of] hope is the means by which it gets there. Second he claims that hope is objective – and thus… public. It does not have to do with our own private agendas… Ultimately hope is divine energy and intelligence loving toward the accomplishment of its purposes: it makes use of us rather than we of it.

– Cynthia Bourgeault

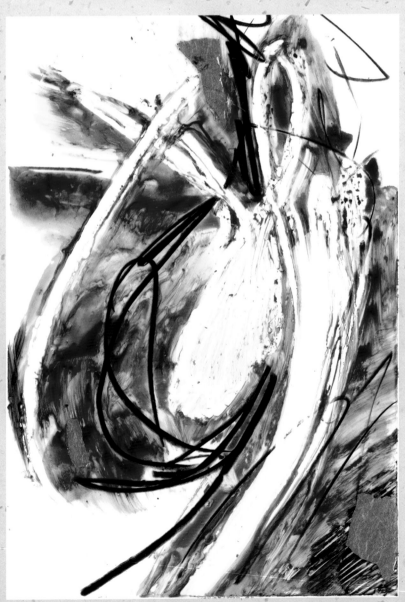

lective birthright. Life on this planet is, in its purest state, erotic – life force animating matter, matter manifesting life force.

The book you hold in your hands is offered into the hope and promise of an emerging sexual-spiritual "third age," wherein the gorgeous symbiotic relationship of spirit and matter is celebrated. In Chapter 1, we find ourselves in the sacred garden that is human sexuality. Chapter 2 recounts the story of our growing human awareness by visiting the sexual-spiritual beliefs and practices of many world traditions. Knowing our story can encourage us to reclaim the good that has been lost, let go of what no longer serves Life, and empower us to embrace our birthright as whole people. Chapters 3 and 4 ask us to "cocoon" into care-full exploration of what it means to be female and male spiritual-sexual beings, touching on some of the challenge, potential, and joy of each. Chapters 5, 6, and 7 – on sensuality, intimacy, and joy, respectively – all offer en*courage*-ment to continue stretching our wings even as we are being transformed. To paraphrase Carl Jung: To be on the journey is to be at the destination. The conclusion offers an inspired vision of the healing power of the erotic spirit, not only for human beings, but for the whole of creation.

As you proceed through the *Spirituality of Sex* you'll be seeing the visions of many artists and photographers, and hearing the thoughts of many past and current sages. You'll notice soon enough that the four of us who've co-authored the book have made no attempt to standardize our voices – choosing rather to offer multiple perspectives and approaches to this vast topic. Further to this end, you'll find a comparable number of woman-authored and man-authored sections in order that the very syntax of the writing as well as its content reflects male and female sensibilities.

May our shared conversation here and beyond serve Life as we continue to heal and grow into our potential as sacred, embodied, and ecstatic human beings. In the economy of Love – as with Grace – nothing is ever wasted. Each incremental act of healing, reconciliation, and integration serves everyone and everything in the seamless Unity.

Sexuality, approached openly, honestly, and with respect for self and other, is not just one of humanity's major evolutionary drives and a possibility for great mental and physical pleasure.

Its function also is to be a most powerful and pleasant means to discover one's inner self, exorcise one's demons, and develop one's potential – in loving communication and cooperation with others.

– *The Encyclopedia of Erotic Wisdom*

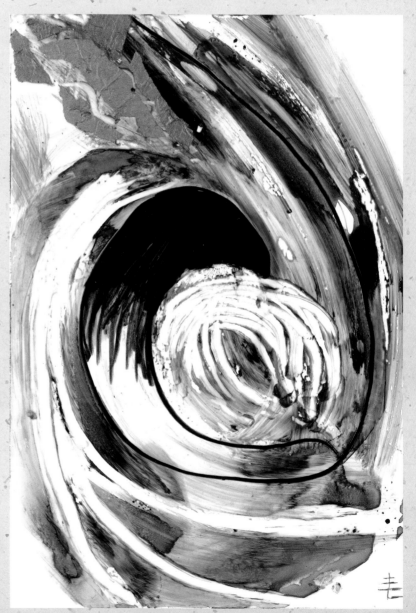

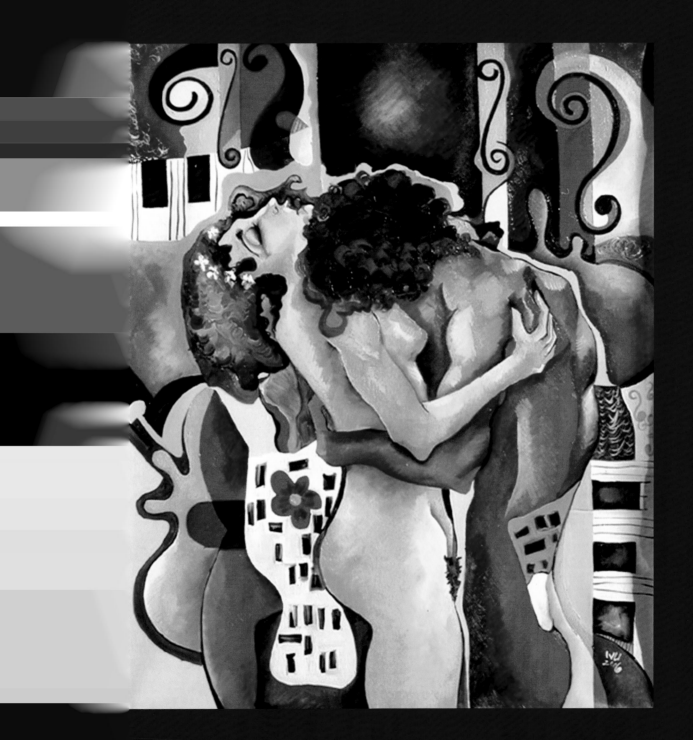

1
The Spirituality of Sex

Michael Schwartzentruber

The body is the spirit incognito.
~ Sandor McNab

We are not human beings trying to become more spiritual.
We are spiritual beings trying to become more human.
~ Teilhard de Chardin

This book is about the spirituality *of* sex. Note that I didn't say spirituality *and* sex, as if sex and spirituality are two unrelated things we might somehow bring together. That little word "of" is important, because it implies that sex and spirituality are intimately related, perhaps even intrinsically, inextricably so.

This is not a new idea, of course, but it hasn't received much attention until relatively recently. Rather, most of us in the West have been raised with the idea that a deep chasm separates sex and spirituality. We've been taught to see sex as a stumbling block, as an obstacle we must overcome if want to realize our true spiritual potential.

Certainly the early apostles and theologians of the Christian tradition – such as Paul and Augustine – played a pivotal role in propagating this notion, and we'll look at some of their ideas more closely in the next chapter. But dusty old theologians aren't

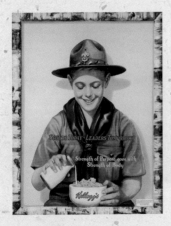

the only ones who have been deeply suspicious and fearful of sex. For example, in the late 1800s, the pseudo-science of men like Sylvester Graham and Dr. John Harvey Kellogg contributed to a general paranoia about the ill effects of masturbation. In fact, graham crackers and Kellogg's Cornflakes were specifically designed to discourage masturbation, on the theory that bland foods dampen the sexual appetites. In a similar vein, the Boy Scout manual went through 57 printings and well into the 1960s con-

taining dire warnings against the perils of masturbation.

One could easily cite hundreds more examples – many books have been written on this topic alone. Suffice it for now to say that for at least the past 2000 years most people in the West have been taught that there is something wrong with sex, and that to be truly spiritual they must somehow rise above, if not repress altogether, their sexual needs and desires.

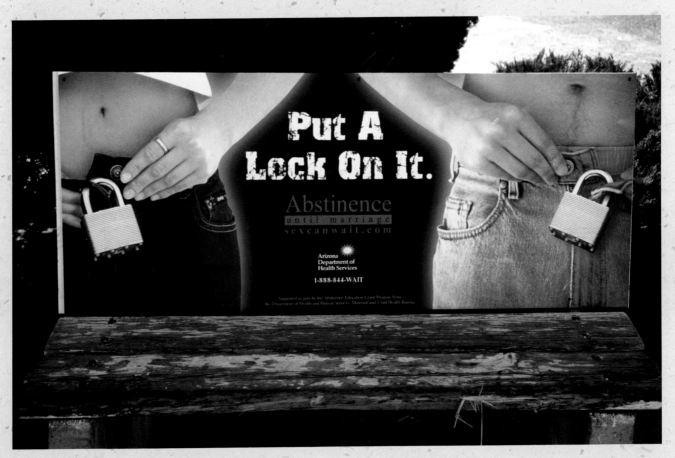

AND IT WAS GOOD…

In this book, we embrace a more holistic possibility, though it is no less ancient – in fact, it is far older – and no less steeped in religious and spiritual tradition. This tradition honours the body and all physical existence as a gift *from* and expression *of* the creative Spirit of God.

In the beginning, says the ancient Hebrew scripture, "God created the heavens and the earth." And God declared it good.

"Then God said, 'Let us make humankind in our image…' So God created humankind *in God's image… male and female* God created *them*" (Genesis 1:26–27).

And God declared it *very good*.

According to this ancient Jewish tradition, sexuality is intrinsic to our humanity. Moreover, we are, in our full humanity, an image or an expression of the divine. Theologians have a fancy word for this idea: they call it *incarnation*.

If the spirituality of sex we present here has a starting point, that's it – our bodies are good and our sexuality is good. Both are a manifestation or incarnation of the divine, and of a divine way of *being*.

There's more to it, of course. A writer I know once said that *spirituality* is the perfect plastic word, because it can mean whatever one wants it to mean. He meant it as a criticism, as a commentary on the fakes and flakiness one sometimes finds on the spiritual fringe. So it's important to say more, to ground this a bit and to be clear about the values, perspectives, and assumptions we bring to this book. Some of those assumptions have to do with the nature and purpose of spirituality. Others have to do with the centrality of relationship, the role of love and lust, the recognition of beauty, the formation of identity, and ultimately the place of sex in the drama of life and death itself. Spiritual stuff indeed.

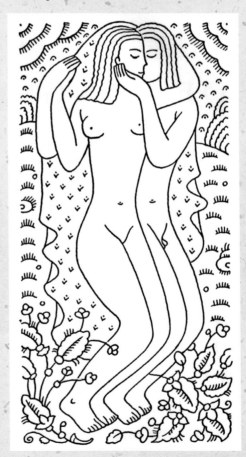

So what exactly are we talking about when we use the word spirituality? I like the quotation from Teilhard de Chardin, which opens the chapter, because it implies that one of the things we acquire as we mature spiritually is a greater sense of our humanness. To this I would add the idea that, at its best, spirituality also makes us more *humane*.

It follows, for me, that what we are talking about when we speak of the spirituality of sex has partly to do with honouring and celebrating our sexual nature, and partly to do with ensuring that the way we *express* our sexuality, including the way we respond to the sexuality of *others*, is as *humane* – as life-enhancing and as life-giving – as possible.

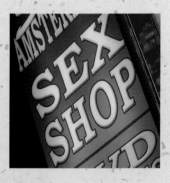

This is an important point, because we live in a culture that tends to treat sex not as something sacred, not as something filled with spiritual energy, but as a commodity, as something external to us that we can buy and sell in a myriad different ways with minimal consequence. We objectify sex. We treat it superficially as a lure. Sex sells, as they say in advertising, and these days we exploit it to sell just about everything.

We also use sex as a weapon, as a means of displaying power in abusive relationships or in times of war, when rape and sexual cruelty seem to know no limits.

On the religious, social, and political fronts, society continues to debate issues related to sexual orientation and same-sex unions, while in many places gay, lesbian, bisexual, and transgendered people suffer unfair treatment, ostracism, and worse.

Beyond all this, many of us know from our own personal histories, or from the histories of those close to us, that not all of our sexual experiences are positive. Which is not to say that these experiences are any less filled with spiritual significance. As Thomas Moore writes in *The Soul of Sex*, "Even if sex is loveless, empty, or manipulative, still it has strong repercussions in the soul, and even bad experiences leave lasting, haunting impressions."[1]

Because of all this, it is important to approach sex wisely. As monk Bede Griffiths once said, "Sex is too powerful a force to deny or put aside on the one hand; but it is also too powerful a force to let run our lives on the other."[2]

We need to keep sex human, and humane.

It Happens All the Time in Heaven

It happens all the time in heaven,
And some day

It will begin to happen
Again on earth –

That men and women who are married,
And men and men who are
Lovers,

And women and women
Who give each other
Light,

Often will get down on their knees

And while so tenderly
Holding their lover's hand,

With tears in their eyes,
Will sincerely speak, saying,

"My dear,
How can I be more loving to you;

How can I become more kind?"

- Hafiz[3] (c. 1320–1389 CE)

LOVE

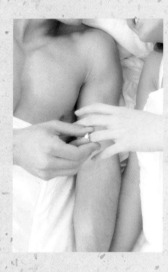

One of the ways we keep sex both human and humane is by wrapping it in the warm and healing blanket called love – an old idea that, in some circles at least, has become new again.

For generations, the only culturally sanctioned or socially acceptable context for sex was within the bounds of a loving, heterosexual marriage relationship. These values worked their way by both direct and subtle means into all levels and spheres of life, to the point that they were ubiquitous and, for many, entirely unconscious.

In the neighbourhood where I grew up, if a boy and a girl (let's call them Peter and Susan) showed any interest in each other, the other kids on the block would torment them with this little chant:

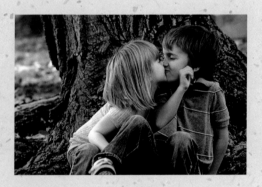

Peter and Susan
sitting in a tree,
K-I-S-S-I-N-G.

First comes love,
then comes marriage,
then comes Susan
with a baby carriage.

As a seven-year-old, I'm pretty sure I had no idea why I joined in – other than that I enjoyed the embarrassment it caused – or how I even came to know such things. But

I did. And so did everybody else. First you fell in love, then you got married, and finally you got to do that thing called "sex." Babies were the result.

But even as I absorbed this old lesson by osmosis, the world was changing. It was the mid-1960s, and the sexual, scientific, and religious revolutions that defined that decade were well underway. Not only were marriage and babies becoming optional, so was love.

In fact, "free love" – the euphemism the '60s used for sex freed from religious guilt and pursued simply for the pleasure of it – proved a misnomer. As Sam Keen writes in his book *The Passionate Life*, love was one of the very *first* things we lost during the sexual revolution.

First, love and sex… were separated. Love became a private, subjective emotion… it was not considered a way of *knowing*… Sex was reduced to a biological phenomenon that scientists could quantify and study objectively in the laboratory… Sensation was divorced from feeling and expectation. Thus liberated, sex became a game, a sport…the well-trained sexual athlete the new model.[4]

At the same time, and in total contradiction to this "stripping away" process, sex

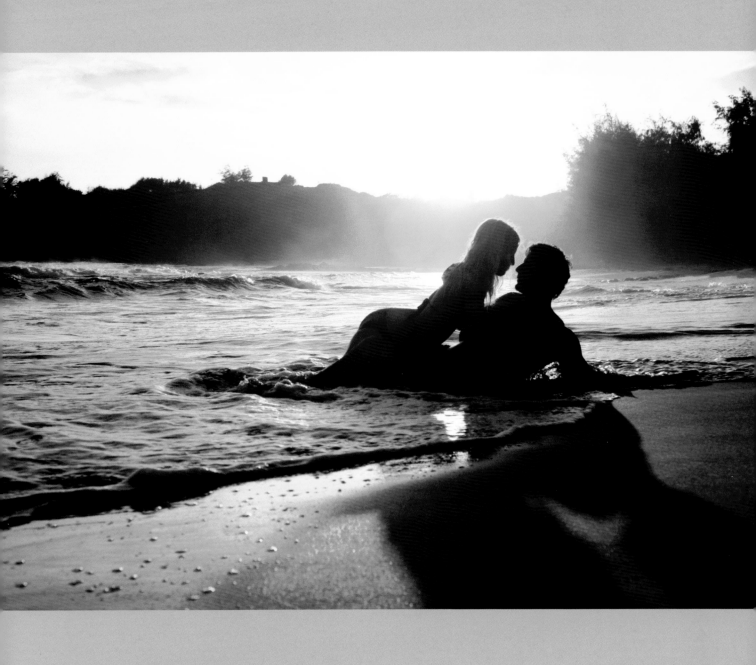

was somehow not only supposed to provide pleasure, it was also supposed to give *meaning* to life. Ultimately, says Keen, the psychic conflict became too much to bear.

Why, we wondered, doesn't this thing we have stripped of awe and made trivial provide us with a center? Liberated sex drove us almost as crazy as the old puritanical kind. One portrayed sex as the devil, the other as God; one promised happiness if we abstained, the other if we indulged. Both lied.[5]

The proof is in the pudding, as they say. While sex without love or emotional investment or commitment may hold a certain appeal (for some) in the short term, I have yet to talk to anyone who has been stuck in that place who hasn't longed to experience sex with an emotionally available and loving partner, or who, having found such a partner, would ever go back to loveless sex.

Put in the simplest terms possible, sex is better when served with a generous helping of love. As Keen writes, "The touch that heals always feels and cherishes the other as a unique human person. It includes the implicit promise of friendship, care, and respect."[6] I take this as a good working definition of love.

Again, this doesn't mean that a loveless one-night stand can't be a spiritual experience or have spiritual significance. If we are

You must not force sex to do the work of love or love to do the work of sex.
~ Mary McCarthy

Only the united beat of sex and heart together can create ecstasy.
~ Anaïs Nin

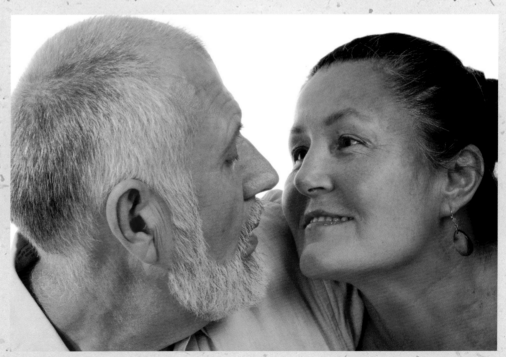

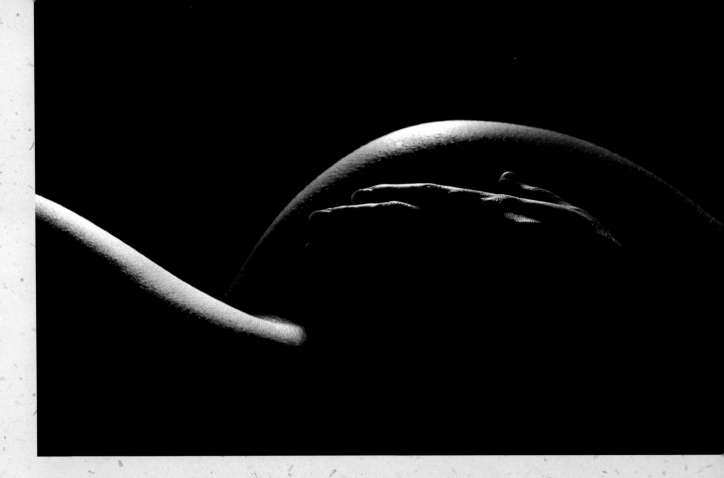

spiritual beings by nature, then *everything* we do has spiritual significance. But experience teaches that the kind of sex that enlivens and deepens us happens most frequently within the context of a loving relationship.

Having said that, I should also say that we have no desire to resurrect in this book the social mores I chanted as a child. In other words, love may come first – it may be the most important thing – but we don't assume here that one has to be married to enjoy this kind of relationship and this kind of sex. We do assume, however, that the best sex happens within some kind of committed, long-term, loving relationship. It takes time and *trust* (an integral part of any love relationship) to plumb the sexual depths of another, to map their erotic body, to discover their desires and explore their fantasies – in short, to learn both the delights they offer and the delights they passionately desire.

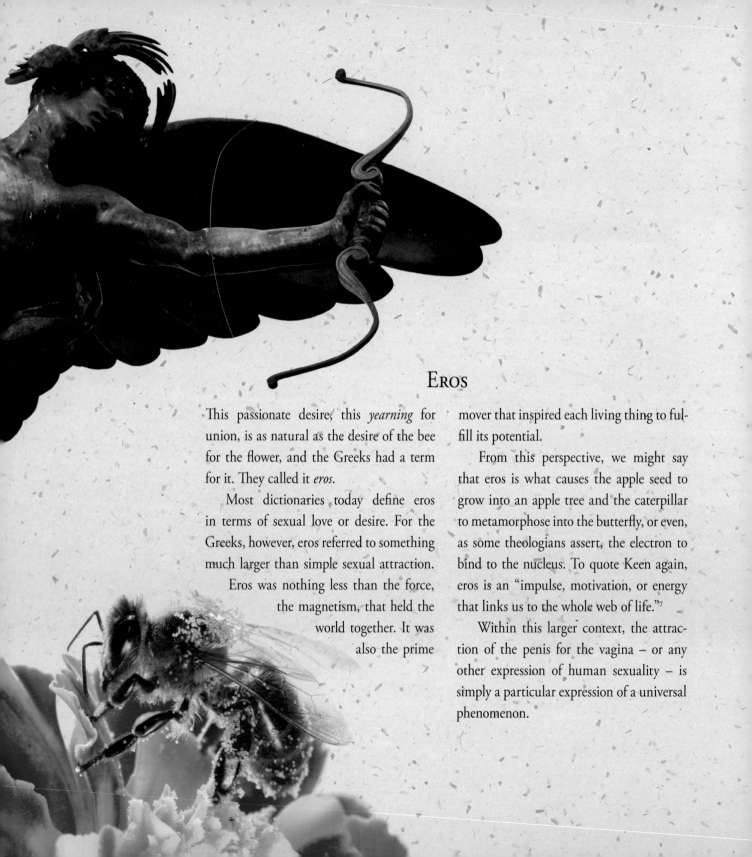

EROS

This passionate desire, this *yearning* for union, is as natural as the desire of the bee for the flower, and the Greeks had a term for it. They called it *eros*.

Most dictionaries today define eros in terms of sexual love or desire. For the Greeks, however, eros referred to something much larger than simple sexual attraction.

Eros was nothing less than the force, the magnetism, that held the world together. It was also the prime mover that inspired each living thing to fulfill its potential.

From this perspective, we might say that eros is what causes the apple seed to grow into an apple tree and the caterpillar to metamorphose into the butterfly, or even, as some theologians assert, the electron to bind to the nucleus. To quote Keen again, eros is an "impulse, motivation, or energy that links us to the whole web of life."[7]

Within this larger context, the attraction of the penis for the vagina – or any other expression of human sexuality – is simply a particular expression of a universal phenomenon.

LUST

If all this sounds just a tad lustful, well, that's good. After all, if it weren't for the lust of our parents and our grandparents and all our ancestors stretching back as far into human history as you care to go, very few of us would actually be here.

And it's not just the lust of our human ancestors we have to thank for our existence. In his book *Sins of the Spirit, Blessings of the Flesh*, Matthew Fox says we should also thank the lust of the animals and birds and insects and fish and flowers and plants and every living thing that makes life on this planet both possible and awe-inspiring. In other words, healthy lust is an expression of the vision of eros, and it is sacred.

We are not used to thinking of lust in this way – as a positive force. Early theologians such as Augustine were no fans of lust and succeeded to an incredible degree in demonizing it, in extinguishing the power of its fire within Western religion and spirituality.

So today, when we think of lust, we usually think of its shadow side, which it certainly has. Lust can go bad, and when it does it looks like violence, addiction, obsession, control, rape, objectification, sexism, abuse, violation, and molestation. "Would we have so many words," asks Fox, "if we did not have the experiences to back them up?"[8]

But none of this is an argument against lust per se. And what would be the point? Lust was, is, and shall be forevermore, amen. Rather, these things remind us that lust, like sex itself, is a powerful force and that sometimes we need to bridle it, or temper it with wisdom and humanity.

But I, for one, would not want to live without lust. Lust in its healthy form is a response to the intensity of the world of the senses and the vibrancy of life. Living lustily is about enjoying the pleasures of the moment to their absolute fullest. When I watch Margaret, my wife, devour a basket of fresh, lusciously red cherries, eyes sparkling, I understand what it means to live lustily. And in that moment she is beautiful, and beautifully alive.

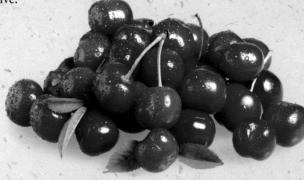

BEAUTY

Love does not recognize the difference between peasant and mikado.

– Japanese proverb

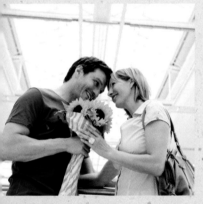

The ability to recognize and appreciate beauty is intrinsic to both healthy spirituality and healthy sexuality, and nowhere is this more significant than in our love relationships. All of us have a deep need to be seen as beautiful, to know ourselves as beautiful. What's more, this beauty is an aspect of the divine. As D. H. Lawrence wrote,

> What's the good of a man unless
>   there's a glimpse of a god in him?
> And what's the good of a woman un-
>   less she's a glimpse of a goddess of
>   some sort?[9]

This is a gift lovers give each other. Lovers see the beauty in each other – both the inner beauty of the soul, and the soul's beauty reflected in the physical body and its actions. It may be a beauty only they can see, but as Thomas Moore says, "even so that beauty is real."[10]

Okay. It's true confessions time. I am a hairy man. It's true. I wish I wasn't, because body hair isn't "in" these days, but I am.

I mention this because Margaret thinks I am beautiful anyway. She loves my body and isn't shy about telling me so. And I need to hear this – that she thinks I am beautiful – because it heals me. It reconnects me to my true self. It restores my soul.

Likewise, when she worries that her hips are too big, or her tummy not flat enough,

she needs to know that I think she is beautiful. And in truth, she is.

"Love is blind." We've all heard it. Maybe we've even said it.

I prefer to believe that love sees with different eyes.

Where deep love and respect are present, there is no such thing as too big or too small, no such thing as not firm enough or flat enough or hard enough. The swell of the breasts, the shape of the buttocks, the form of the physique as seen in the arms, shoulders, torso and thighs – often we know and cherish the beauty of these things in our partners, even when they can't see that beauty themselves.

What's more, lovers have the power to evoke that beauty, particularly the beauty of the face. If you've ever spent time in an airport watching as partners reunite, you know what I mean. In an instant, at the first glimpse of the other, the heart redraws the face. Everything shifts. Stress lines disappear. Eyes sparkle. Lips and mouths soften. Sometimes the transformation is nothing less than miraculous.

This ability of lovers to both recognize and draw forth the beauty of their beloved is precious and needs to be defended against the definitions of beauty promoted by secular culture – definitions that tend to be only skin deep and blind to the vision of beauty that is the special gift of love, intimacy, and respect.

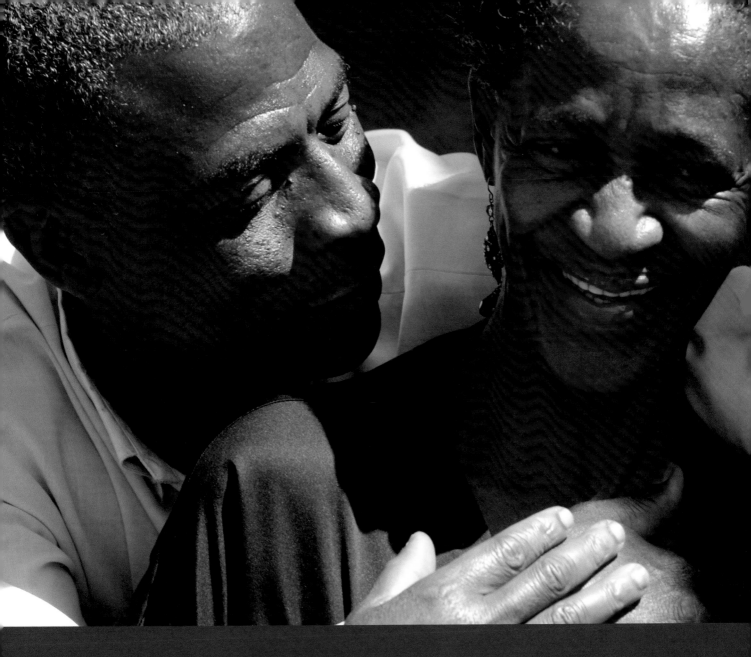

Archetypal human beauty shines through in every body and every face, especially to a lover or a parent, and that beauty, with its seductiveness, is part of the life of the soul.

- THOMAS MOORE

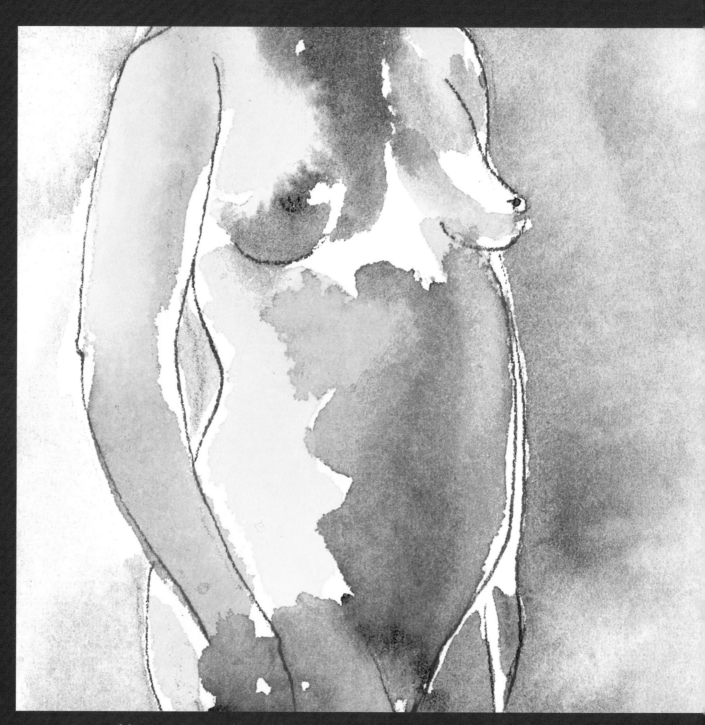

Sex and beauty are one thing, like flame and fire.
If you hate sex, you hate beauty.
If you love living beauty, you have a reverence for sex.
— D. H. LAWRENCE

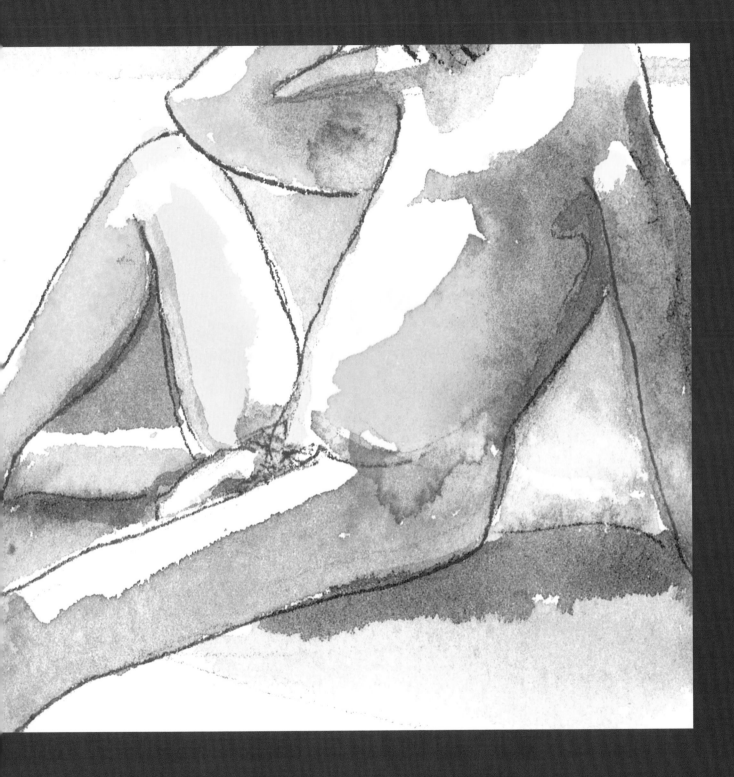

IDENTITY

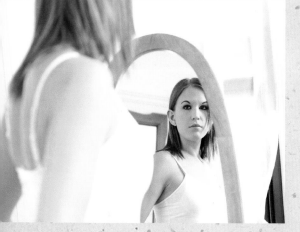

Cultural definitions of beauty and the pressure to conform to "ideal" body types can play havoc with our sense of identity. If you're not happy with your body, it's unlikely you're going to feel good about your "self," your sense of who you are as a person. Most people begin to internalize these pressures during adolescence, typically a time when we become extremely self-conscious and concerned about our looks.

During that same period, something else with even deeper sexual and spiritual implications may be going on, says Robert Bly in *The Maiden King*, a book he co-wrote with Jungian analyst Marion Woodman.

It's not exactly news that adolescence is the time when most of us awaken to the potential of our sexuality. But in many cultures, including our own, adolescence is also a time of spiritual awakening. Each of these awakenings, or openings, is accompanied by a sense of great expectation, as if something wonderful is about to happen. This and the fact that they happen almost simultaneously means that sexuality and spirituality can easily become confused.

In order to properly integrate sexuality and spirituality into our personality, says Bly, each of these awakenings must receive a positive response from the outer world – from parents or other significant adults, or from the culture in general. If this happens, the "corresponding power" becomes integrated into the self. But if the inner awakening *doesn't* receive support from the outside world, then the opposite happens. The opening closes; the window of opportunity is lost to the developing self and the *great expectation* turns into *great disappointment.*

Generally speaking, in North American culture, the spiritual awakening receives very little support from the outside world. Often we're not even aware that it's happening. But the sexual awakening! Everywhere we turn it's all about sex – billboard-size lingerie ads, beauty magazines, movies, music videos and television shows filled with sex and sexual innuendo.

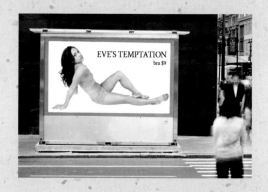

In other words, the spiritual opening is virtually ignored or denied while the sexual opening receives all the attention.

The result is that the American adolescent tries to receive from sexuality the marvellous ecstasy that his or her cells have been promised by the spiritual opening. "It must surely come." But the ecstasy doesn't come. What arrives is disappointment. The adolescent feels horrific despair when the sexual chakra does not deliver the ecstasy that he or she believes will come.[11]

Many people carry this disappointment and confusion their entire lives, endlessly pursuing sex for something that sex alone cannot give. Without spirit, without a point of deep grounding or connection, sex is powerless to save us or to give our lives meaning.

The task of sexual-spiritual integration and identity building is even harder if our sexual orientation or our gender association (our sense of our gender, which may or may not match the genitals we were born with) is held suspect by our culture or faith community.

Finally, of course, the question of identity is directly related to our perception, or not, of ourselves as spiritual beings, which is where we began the chapter.

And so we have come full circle.

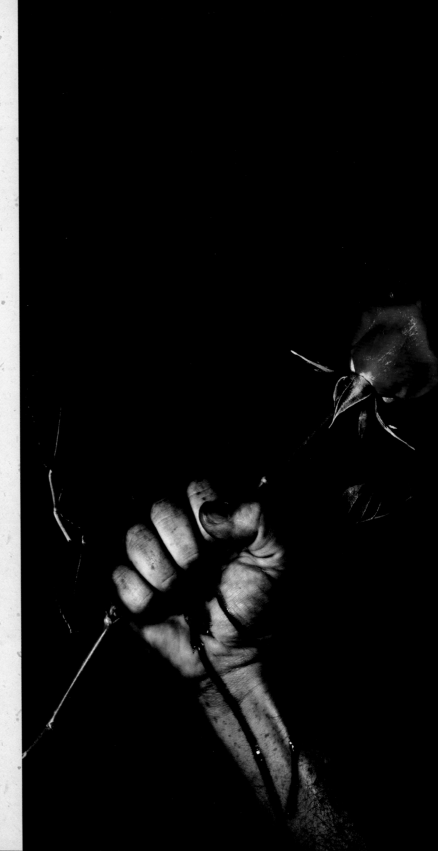

LIFE AND DEATH

But there is a larger circle at play here, too. Ultimately, sex is spiritual because through sex we participate in the greatest of all spiritual mysteries – the circle of life and death. This is true both on a literal and a metaphorical level.

On a purely literal, biological level, sex and death – *eros* and *thanatos* – are inherently linked. Sex is evolution's answer to the problem of death, at least within the plant and animal kingdoms. Every life form is subject to decay and death, and therefore must have a way to reproduce itself. Sex for procreation is thus an integral part of the wheel of life. Without it, the wheel would stop turning and we would cease to be.

Not that we're likely to be thinking about death when we're having sex, especially when we're intentionally trying to make a baby. If anything, the opposite is true. Sex makes us feel vital and alive.

Yet death plays a role in our sexuality in subtle and sometimes not-so-subtle ways, perhaps most significantly at midlife.

Second true confession. Unlike a lot of guys, I enjoy romantic comedies, at least if they're intelligent and well-written. To my mind, *Moonstruck* falls into this category. In the film, Loretta Castorini (played by Cher) is engaged to Johnny Cammareri. Johnny is not her ideal mate, but the grey hairs that have recently begun to frame her face have convinced her that time is running out. So she "settles." But then Johnny goes to Italy to tend to his dying mother. While he's away, Loretta meets Ronny, Johnny's younger brother (played by Nicolas Cage). Ronny is everything Johnny is not. Suffice it to say, Loretta and Ronny discover a passion and a connection that quickly leads to romance, sex, and "true love."

Meanwhile, we discover that Loretta's father, Cosmo, is also in the midst of an affair. Cosmo's wife, Rose (played by Olympia Dukakis), is suspicious.

In my favourite scene, Johnny has just returned home from Italy and goes straight to see Loretta. Loretta's not home because she's out with Ronny. But Rose is home and she needs to talk. She drags Johnny into the living room, gets him seated, and then puts the question to him: "Why do men chase women?"

At first, Johnny misunderstands the question and replies that perhaps a man needs a woman in order to be whole.

Exasperated, Rose asks, "Why would a man need more than one woman?"

Johnny shrugs. "I don't know. Maybe because he fears death?"

"That's it!" Rose cries.

At exactly that moment, Cosmo – who has just been to the opera with the "other" woman – walks in the door.

"Where have you been?" demands Rose.

"I don't know, Rose. I don't know where I've been; I don't know where I'm going." Wearily, as if carrying the weight of the world, he starts climbing the stairs.

"Cosmo," says Rose sternly, fixing him in place with her stare, "I just want you to know, it doesn't matter what you do, you're going to die."

I love that scene both for its humour and for its deep wisdom. How many people have fallen, either consciously or unconsciously, into an affair at midlife because they have an uneasy sense that time might be running out on them, or because they somehow experience themselves to be less than they used to be, or because they want to make a change and it seems like

it's now or never? And what are all of these things if not intimations of mortality?

In the face of this, the power of the romantic affair is precisely the rekindling of passion and the sense of vitality and new life it can inspire. Sometimes these things will be better sought from the original relationship; sometimes not. But that's not the point. The point is, we often turn to sex and perhaps even more so to romantic love in our struggle to come to grips with our mortality.

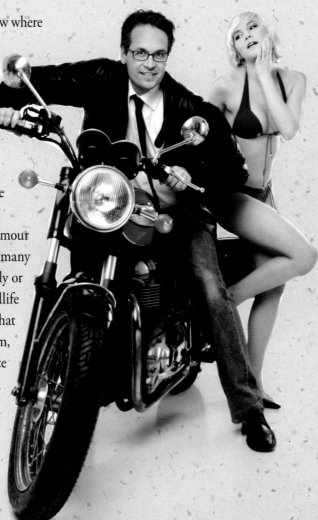

La Petite Mort and Mystical Sex

Sex and death are also linked in less literal, more metaphorical ways. *La petite mort* – the little death – is a French phrase that originally referred to the tendency of some women (and a proportionately smaller number of men) to pass out during orgasm. Today we use it to refer to orgasm in general.

Quite aside from all of this, I like the phrase because, to my mind at least, it conveys a very real spiritual truth. There is a

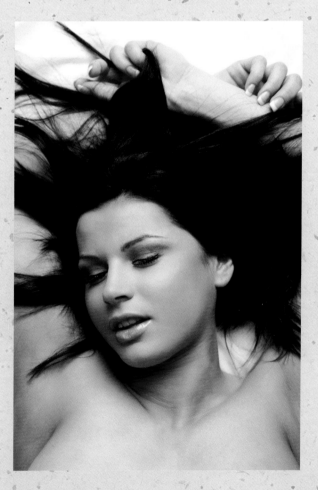

sense in which we *do* die to our "selves" or "lose ourselves" during sex – particularly during orgasm.

We know, for instance, that our ability to process sense information during sex and orgasm declines drastically. If you've ever been "caught in the act" because you failed to hear someone (a child perhaps) call out your name, or climb the stairs, or open the door, you'll know exactly what I mean.

On a more profound level, we also die to our "selves" in that very few of us are able to maintain our inhibitions and psychic masks during orgasm. Even more than being physically naked, we are psychically and spiritually naked. Some people laugh during orgasm, some weep, some cry out. Whatever the response, surely it comes from a place deep inside of us and expresses something of the soul.

We can go deeper still. As an individual, I can also die to myself or lose myself when I give myself over completely to my partner. When both partners do this, give themselves over to the other completely, they may experience a sense of oneness. At its pinnacle, this may include not only a sense of oneness with each other, but a sense of oneness with all of life and even with God. What we're talking about here is the mystical potential of sex – sex as a transcendent, unifying experience.

AND STILL THERE'S MORE

I started down this path of talking about relationships, and love, and eros, and lust, and beauty, and identity, and life and death because I said that when it comes to the spirituality of sex, there's more to say than simply "sex is spiritual." I wanted to set out some of our underlying assumptions and understandings.

Having done that, I'm aware that there is *still* more to be said – much more – about all of these things. That "more" is what the rest of this book is about.

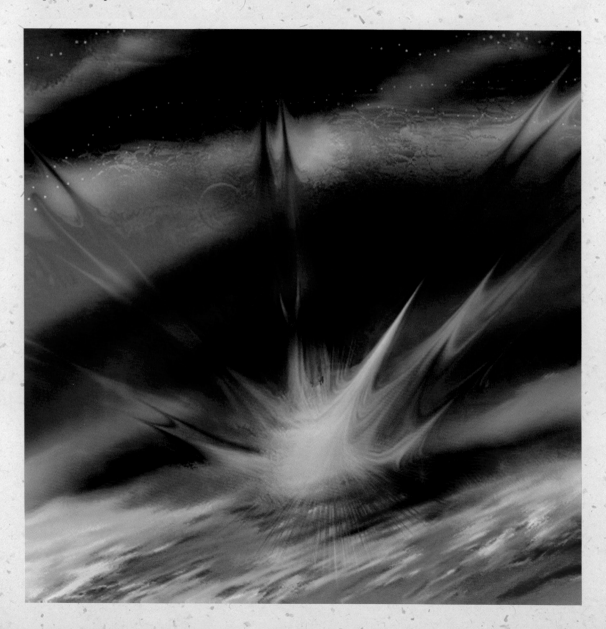

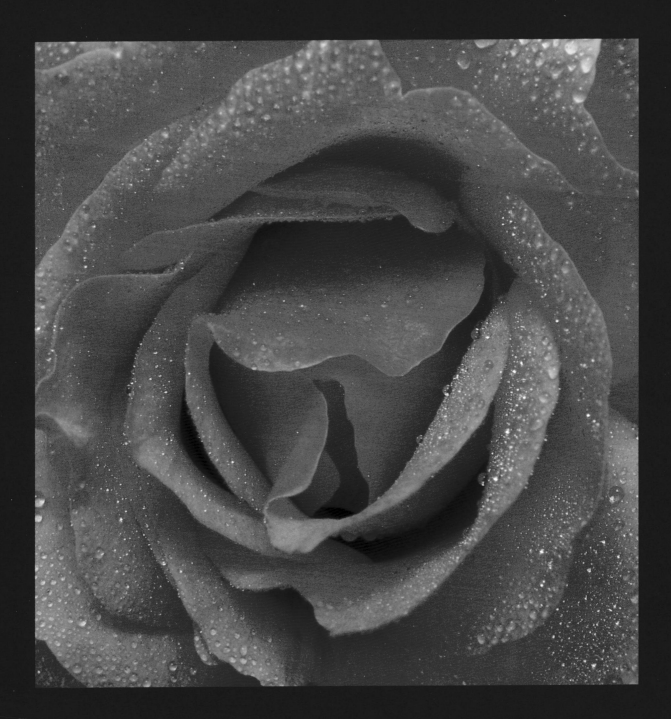

2
Religion and the Erotic Spirit

MICHAEL SCHWARTZENTRUBER

Spirituality must be sexual if it is to be human spirituality.
We love God either as ensexed and embodied creatures or not at all.
We love God as humans who are men and women all the time in
everything we do.

~ DODY H. DONNELLY, *RADICAL LOVE*

Like a great many people, I grew up believing that religion and sex don't mix. The idea has been embedded in our cultural and religious landscape for such a long time, I think I simply absorbed it by osmosis. Even so, I count myself lucky. Many people have had the idea driven home by religious parents or teachers who preached hell-fire and brimstone for sexual "misbehaviours" of all sorts. Depending on their home or school situation, everything from showing their "private parts" or playing "doctor" as children, to kissing, masturbation, and pre-marital sex was deemed dirty or sinful and was grounds for punishment.

I was fortunate to escape this kind of heavy-handed repression. Nevertheless, I found it liberating to discover that not all religions held the same negative view of sex as mine seemed to do. I was even more intrigued to learn that there is an erotic thread that runs through almost all religious traditions, including my own Christian tradition.

In truth, as a species, we have been trying to figure out sex for a very, *very* long time. Sex is powerful stuff, after all, a veritable force of nature. And so, since the dawn of human history, we have tried to place it in the largest possible context, to understand what it means in terms of our experience of life and of the sacred power that animates it.

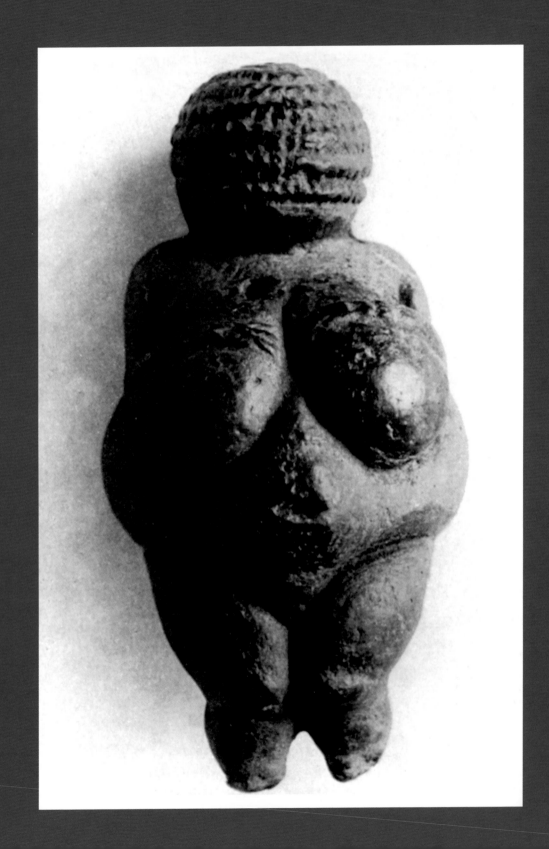

Our first conscious attempts to get hold of sex in this larger sense appear to have begun as far back as 25,000 to 30,000 years ago, when our Stone Age ancestors began drawing female symbols on cave walls, and carving statuettes of the female form out of stone, bone, and other materials. Typically, these statuettes show a woman with huge breasts, broad hips, and often a clearly discernable vulva.

Although no one can know for sure, some scholars believe that these figures represent the original Great Mother or Earth Mother. Because at this very early date people had not yet made the connection between sexual intercourse and procreation, this Great Mother may have been seen as the sole source of life. And not just of human life, but of all animal and plant life, too. As a representation of this Goddess or Ancestress, the statuettes may have been used in early fertility rituals.

In time, the discovery that males played a part in making babies led to an array of beliefs and rituals that celebrated and linked in a magical way the sexual intercourse of the gods, human sexual intercourse, the cycle of the seasons, the fertility of the soil, and the success of crops.

One of those rituals was the annual *hieros gamos*, or sacred marriage rite. This ritual is first mentioned in Sumerian texts dating from about 3,000 BCE, but had probably been around long before then.

By this time (at least 20,000 years after those first figures were carved), the Goddess was no longer a generic Earth Mother figure. Each culture where she was found gave her a name and a personal history. Thus, says Georg Feuerstein in his book *Sacred Sexuality*, she was "Inanna in Sumer, Ishtar in Babylon, Anath in Canaan, Astarte in Phoenicia, Isis in Egypt, Nu Kua in China, Freya in Scandinavia, and Kunapipi in aboriginal Australia."[1] And because people now knew that males played a role in procreation, she was also joined by a male deity who was her lover.

In the *hieros gamos* ritual, a human couple – perhaps the chief priestess and chief priest, or the queen and her male consort – re-enacted the sexual intercourse of the Goddess and her divine male partner. In doing so, they were not just playing a role. Rather, both male and female participants believed that they were incarnating the God and Goddess and the life force each represented. To the degree the participants were able to experience this, the *hieros gamos* was about self-transcendence.

Though no one knows exactly how the ritual was performed, an ancient Sumerian hymn, which was probably recited during the ritual, reveals its erotic nature. In the excerpt that follows, the Goddess Inanna and the divine Dumuzi address each other.

My vulva, the horn,
The Boat of Heaven,
Is full of eagerness like the young
    moon.
My untilled land lies fallow.

As for me Inanna,
Who will plough my vulva?
Who will plough my high field?
Who will plough my wet ground?

As for me, the young woman
Who will plough my vulva?
Who will station the ox there?
Who will plough my vulva?

Great Lady, the king will plough your
    vulva.
I, Dumuzi, will plough your vulva.

Then plough my vulva, man of my
    heart!
Plough my vulva![2]

The important thing to know about all of this is that, in these very early times, our ancestors understood that the entire cosmos, including sexuality, was a manifestation or expression of sacred power or the sacred life force. The dualistic categories of sacred and profane, which lead to guilt and shame, did not exist. Rituals such as the *heiros gamos* were one way in which they sought to manipulate, for their own well-being, as well as celebrate and share this sacred life force.

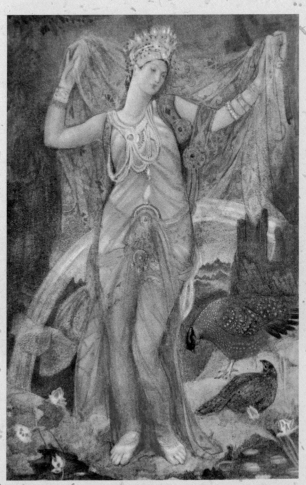

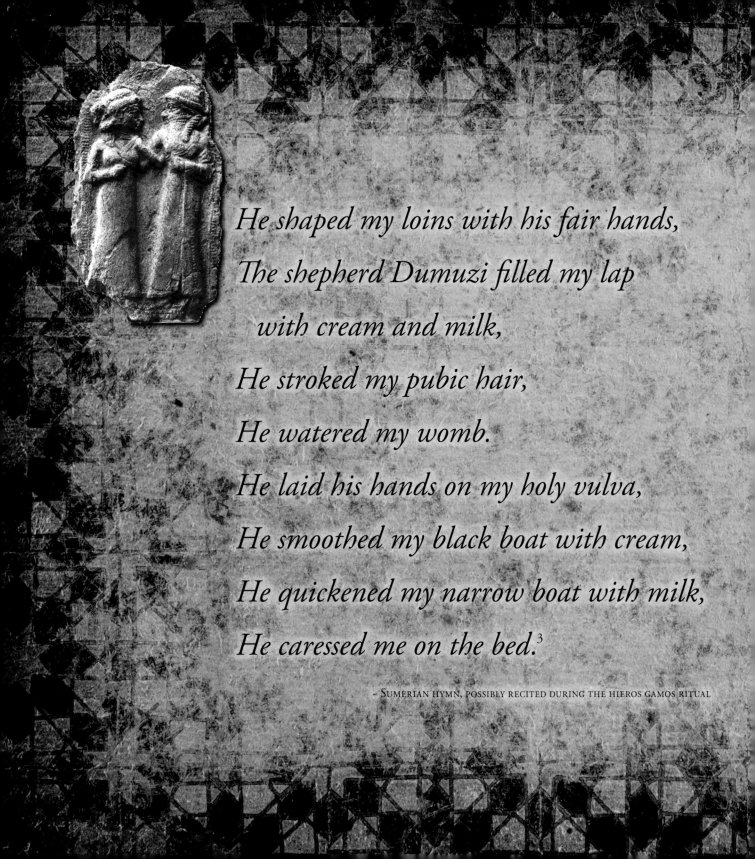

He shaped my loins with his fair hands,

The shepherd Dumuzi filled my lap

with cream and milk,

He stroked my pubic hair,

He watered my womb.

He laid his hands on my holy vulva,

He smoothed my black boat with cream,

He quickened my narrow boat with milk,

He caressed me on the bed.[3]

~ SUMERIAN HYMN, POSSIBLY RECITED DURING THE HIEROS GAMOS RITUAL

THE RISE OF THE PHALLUS AND PATRIARCHY

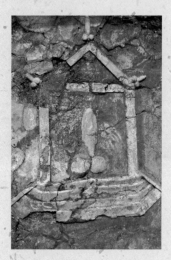

Although the Goddess and her divine male consort managed to live together amicably for a time, in the end, the discovery that men played a role in sexual reproduction spelled disaster for their relationship.

It didn't take long before men claimed that it was *their* semen, their seed, that planted life in the female, and that the woman's role was merely to nourish it and protect it in her womb (a view that only began to be questioned in the mid-1600s with the rise of Western science, and that was only finally disproved in 1827 when the first human ovum was seen with a microscope).[4] Soon the tradition of the Goddess came under systematic attack. Women and female sexuality were subjugated as male domination and the force of patriarchy grew and spread.

As religious thought began to shift more and more towards the power and influence of male deities, the phallus grew in importance in many cultures. Nowhere was this more evident than in ancient Greece and Rome, where the phallus was prominently displayed in artwork and adorned everything from inscriptions to paving stones to doorways.

It's important to note here that in terms of its spiritual or religious or symbolic meaning, a phallus is not the same thing as a real-life penis. And although today we tend to think that phallic symbols represent the male ego, in ancient times they represented fertility, just like those statuettes of the Goddess and the representations of the vulva found on cave walls. In Roman times, the phallus also represented prosperity and abundance, as well as sexual pleasure – in other words, all the things of a good and full life.

These themes can be seen in a painting that once hung in the House of the Vettii, in Pompeii. This painting depicts the god Priapus, his huge member resting on one side of a weigh scale, a bag of coins balanced on the other, and below the scale a cornucopia of fruit.

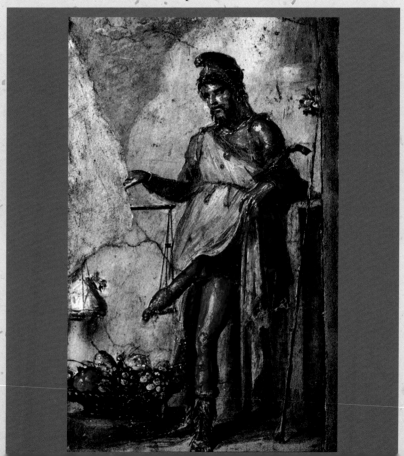

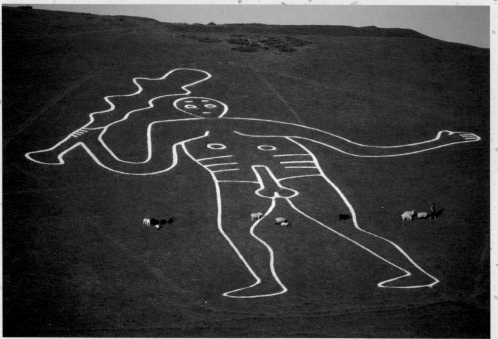

Given the weight of meaning the phallus carried, it's not surprising that ancient depictions of it were often larger than life. The phallus on the Cerne Abbas Giant, for example, located in Dorset, England, is 26 feet long.

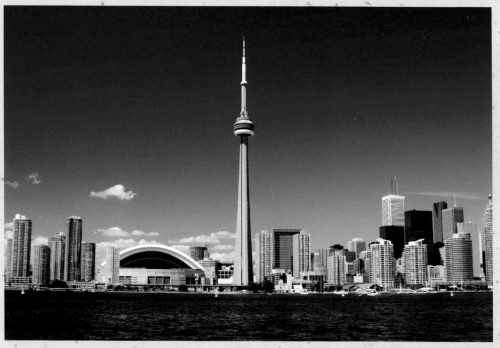

In many ways, modern culture is just as phallocentric as ancient cultures were; our symbols are just less explicitly sexual. Instead of drawing, painting, and sculpting penises, we erect skyscrapers and towers, symbols of wealth, power, and domination.

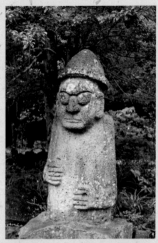

According to Thomas Moore, the phallus is "a representation of earth's potency and life's capacity for creativity and pleasure." The phallus "represents life itself – procreative, pleasurable, rising and falling, penetrating, healing, enduring."[5]

If only our ancestors could have found a way to honour these phallic virtues without at the same time denigrating women and female sexuality. As it turned out, of course, patriarchy gave men great power to define what would, in each culture, constitute "acceptable" forms of sexual expression, especially in relation to the divine – with a great variety of results.

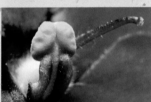

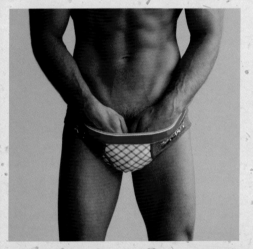

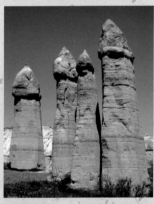

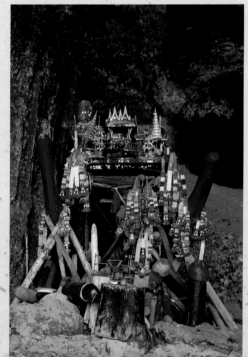

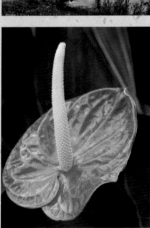

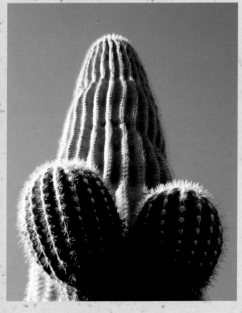

The Erotic Spirit in Judaism

We don't usually think of the Jewish religion as being particularly erotic or even sex-positive. Ancient Judaism was, after all, strongly patriarchal: women were considered "chattel," or property, and many of the laws of ancient Israel seem designed to restrict and control female sexuality for the benefit of men. Still, the Hebrew scriptures show that the ancient Jews also appreciated the goodness of human sexuality and the joy sex can bring.

In Chapter 1, I mentioned the Jewish creation myth in which humans – male and female alike – are created in the image of God (Genesis 1:27). This seminal story recognizes the goodness inherent in the sexuality of both men and women – a pretty abstract theological idea, to be sure.

But the Jews were also great pragmatists. Because producing children was extremely important to them, they honoured and took measures to protect the role of procreation and sex in marriage. Deuteronomy 24:5, for example, declares,

> When a man is newly married, he shall not go out with the army or be charged with any related duty. He shall be free at home one year, to be happy with the wife whom he has married.

Likewise, Proverbs 5:15–19 honours the role of sex, love, and fidelity in marriage (of both male and female partners), in beautifully metaphoric and fairly explicit terms.

> Drink water from your own cistern, flowing water from your own well.
> Should your springs be scattered abroad, streams of water in the streets?
> Let them be for yourself alone, and not for sharing with strangers.
> Let your fountain be blessed, and rejoice in the wife of your youth, a lovely deer, a graceful doe.
> May her breasts satisfy you at all times; may you be intoxicated always by her love.

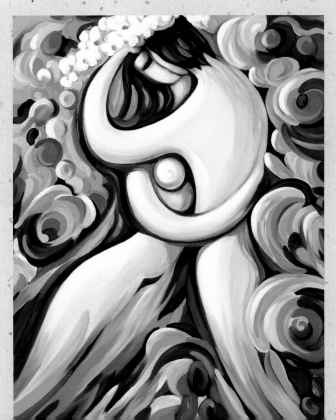

But we find the most obvious example of the erotic spirit in ancient Judaism in the collection of love poems known as the Song of Songs (or the Song of Solomon). In the selection below (4:10–16), the two lovers address each other as brother/sister, but also as bride and beloved.

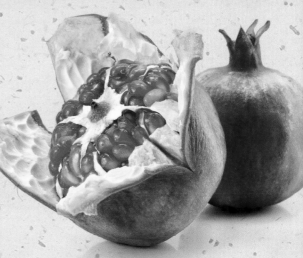

How sweet is your love, my sister, my bride!
  how much better is your love than wine,
   and the fragrance of your oils than any spice!
Your lips distill nectar, my bride;
  honey and milk are under your tongue;
   the scent of your garments is like the scent of Lebanon.
A garden locked is my sister, my bride,
  a garden locked, a fountain sealed.
Your channel is an orchard of pomegranates
  with all choicest fruits, henna with nard,
   nard and saffron, calamus and cinnamon…
a garden fountain, a well of living water,
  and flowing streams from Lebanon.

[The woman replies]
Awake, O north wind,
  and come, O south wind!
Blow upon my garden
  that its fragrance my be wafted abroad.
Let my beloved come to his garden,
  and eat its choicest fruits.

The highly suggestive metaphors used here make this erotic, sensual stuff indeed. The male lover, for example, describes the "channel" of his beloved as an orchard of pomegranates, traditionally one of the most erotic of fruits, with its luscious, red interior. Professor of religion Teresa J. Hornsby notes that when the woman is sexually aroused, "her waters flow like a stream out of Lebanon." She is a "garden fountain, a well of living water."[6]

Hornsby also notes how the woman entreats the winds to blow upon her "garden," to carry the scent of her sex to her lover so that he may come and eat of her fruit – one of several thinly veiled references to oral sex in the collection of poems as a whole.

No wonder the Jewish priests who compiled the Hebrew canon debated whether to include this work. In the end, they got around the "problem" of its erotic nature by reading it as an allegory or metaphor of the love that exists between Israel and God.

While this may be a perfectly valid interpretation, a more literal reading that understands the Song of Songs as a hymn to human sexual love also has things to teach. Sex between loving partners – married or not (scholars like to point out that the poems don't mention marriage) – is a gift.

Still, the dominant Jewish perspective emphasized both the goodness of sex *and* the importance of marriage. As Georg Feuerstein says,

For the ancient Hebrews, just as for the modern Jews, marriage and sexual relations between husband and wife were a sacrament, and the delight that they give each other in their intimacy was regarded as a *mitzvah*, or a divinely dispensed law.[7]

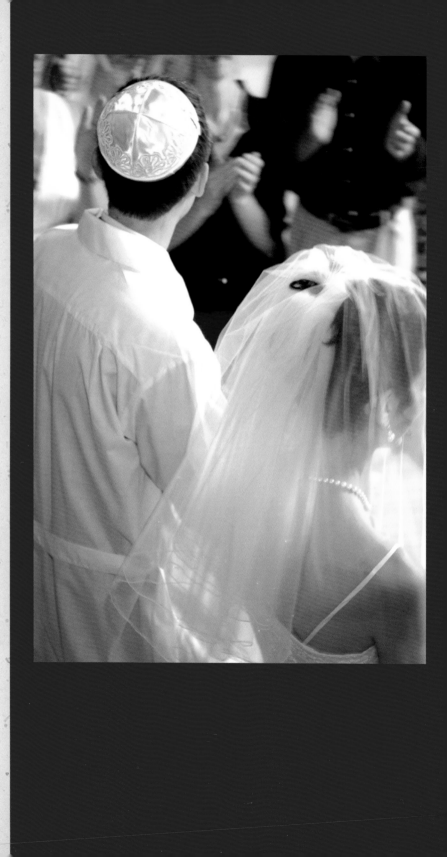

The Christian Love Mystics

While perhaps nothing could seem more natural than sex between husband and wife, from its earliest days Christianity adopted a very cautious stance towards both marriage *and* marital sex.

No doubt one reason for this was the early Christian community's belief in the immanent return of Christ. What's the point of marriage, after all, if you think life as you know it is about to end? As the apostle Paul recommended, better to remain spiritually focused and therefore spiritually prepared for what's to come by staying single and celibate (1 Corinthians 7:1–39).

This early caution around sex grew more negative under the influence of St. Augustine (354–430 CE), one of the "founding fathers" of the Christian church. Sexually promiscuous in his a youth, Augustine struggled most of his life to subdue what he thought was the biggest obstacle to his spiritual growth: lust. His feelings of guilt about his former life and his loathing of his own sex drive deeply affected his view of marriage, sex, and women, whom he saw as temptresses. Soon after his conversion to Christianity, he wrote, "I have decided that there is nothing I should avoid so much as marriage. I know nothing which brings the manly mind down from the heights more than a woman's caresses and that joining of bodies without which one cannot have a wife."[8]

Augustine's views on sex reflect a profound disconnect or dualism between matter and spirit, body and soul, women and men. In his view, spirit, soul, and maleness were all related and were all good; while matter, the body, and femaleness were all linked and were all bad.

To be fair, Augustine didn't think up this scenario all by himself. He had help, mostly from Manichean Gnosticism, which held that the universe is composed of two essential natures: light and darkness, which represent good and evil, respectively. According to the Manicheans, each person was a battleground for these powers. In their scheme, the soul (which was good because it was composed of light) was constantly at war with the body (which was bad because it was composed of matter or dark earth).

Unfortunately, Augustine's ideas about sex came to dominate Western Christianity, and therefore Western culture.

The result of this was that asceticism, monasticism, and celibacy all became part of the religious ideal within the Roman Catholic Church, and a requirement for priests and anyone entering the religious life.[9]

But this sexual repression didn't stop at the monastery gates; it was imposed on society as a whole. At every turn, average people were taught that sex was shameful and carried a burden of guilt. Sex, they were told, was for procreation only. At one point, sexual repression became so great that people weren't allowed to have sex on Sundays, Wednesdays, and Fridays; three days before Communion; the 40 days of Lent; and the 40 days before Christmas.

Yet the erotic impulse will find expression one way or another. One of those ways was through the Christian love mystics – people such as Mechthild of Magdeburg, Hildegard of Bingen, Teresa of Avila, and many others. Although celibate, these people gave voice to the union they experienced with God using erotic language and imagery. Mechthild of Magdeburg (c. 1210 – c. 1282 CE) wrote,

How the soul speaks to God
Lord you are my lover,
> My longing,
> My flowing stream,
> My sun,
And I am your reflection.

How God Answers the Soul
It is my nature that makes me love you often,
> For I am love itself.
It is my longing that makes me love you intensely,
> For I yearn to be loved from the heart.
It is my eternity that makes me love you long,
> For I have no end.[10]

Many of these mystics were, in fact, inspired by the language and imagery of the Song of Songs. Thus, Teresa of Avila (1515–1582 CE) wrote,

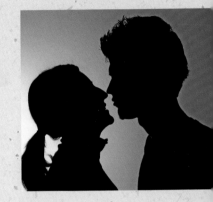

> God and the soul understand each other… It's like the experience of two persons here on earth who love each other deeply and understand each other well; even without signs, just by a glance, it seems, they understand each other… These two lovers gaze directly at each other, as the Bridegroom says to the Bride in the *Song of Songs*.[11]

This type of mysticism – in which God or Christ (the bridegroom) seeks intimate union with the human soul (the bride) – became known as "bridal mysticism."

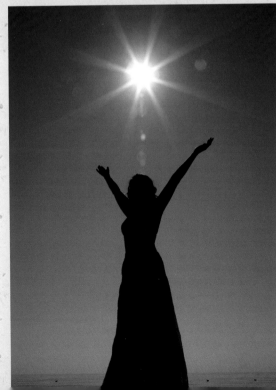

In Bernini's *St. Teresa in Ecstasy*, we see Teresa in the throes of a spiritual ecstasy, which, from the artist's perspective, has clearly sexual, almost orgasmic overtones. The sculpture is based on St. Teresa's description of one of her own mystical experiences.

I saw close to me toward my left side an angel in bodily form… I saw in his hands a large golden dart… It seemed to me this angel plunged the dart several times into my heart and that it reached deep within me. When he drew it out, I thought he was carrying off with him the deepest part of me; and he left me all on fire with great love of God. The pain was so great it made me moan, and the sweetness this greatest pain caused me was so superabundant that there is no desire capable of taking it away; nor is the soul content with less than God… The loving exchange that takes place between the soul and God is so sweet that I beg Him in His goodness to give a taste of this love to anyone who thinks I am lying.[12]

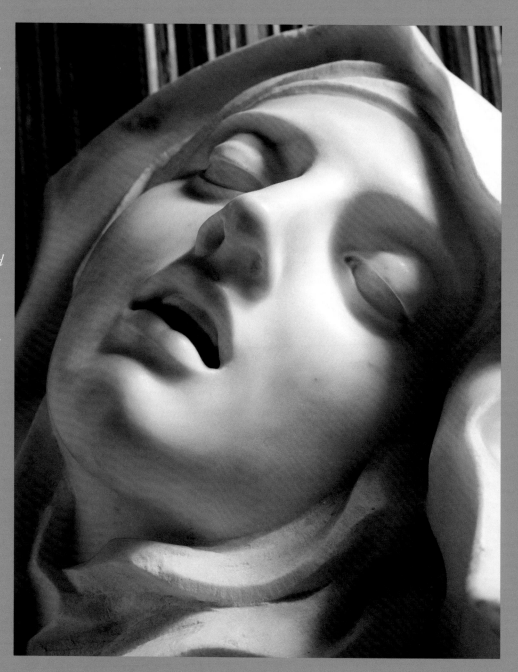

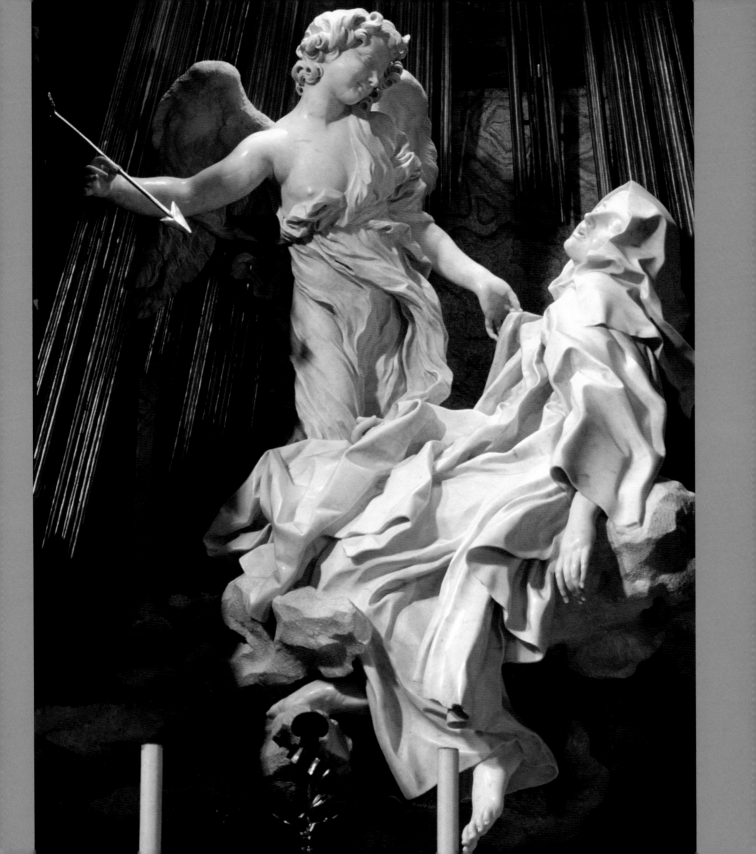

THE JEWISH LOVE MYSTICS

It was not just the medieval Christian mystics who spoke about their relationship with God in this way. During roughly the same period – the 12th to 13th centuries – both Jewish mystics and Sufi mystics in Islam gave voice to their highest spiritual aspirations and most intimate experiences of the divine using erotic language and imagery.

In Judaism, the term *Kabbalah* refers to mystical teachings. The *Zohar*, which was written in the 13th century, is perhaps the most important text of the Kabbalah. According to the *Zohar*, the divine incorporates both male and female elements: "Any image that does not embrace male and female is not a high and true image."[13] In order for there to be harmony in the cosmos, these male and female aspects must be joined or have union (*yihud*):

Come and see:
The blessed Holy One does not place his abode
in any place where male and female are not found together.
Blessings are found only in a place were male and female are found,
A human being is only called Adam When male and female are as one."[14]

What's more, because there is a "perfect parallelism" between the earthly and divine realms, human sexual activity influences what happens in the divine realm. Thus, the sexual pleasure of a human couple is able to magnify the peace in the world.[15]

What a difference between the Kabbalists and the Christian mystics, who tried at every turn to avoid actual sexual relationships! As Feuerstein says,

True to the prominent asceticism of their tradition, the Christian love mystics sought to sublimate the sexual urge without denying eros. By contrast, the much more world-embracing Jewish mystics were not content with cultivating the erotic through allegory and metaphor. Showing perhaps sounder instinct, they embraced their wives while remembering the divine.[16]

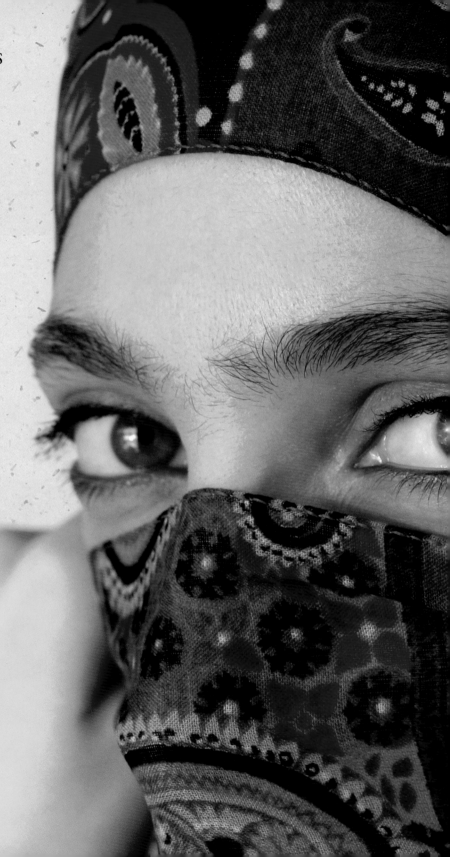

THE SUFI LOVE MYSTICS

The same could also be said about the Sufi mystics, many of whom were married – including perhaps the best-known Sufi mystic and poet of them all, Jalal al-Din Rumi (1207–1273 CE), known today simply as Rumi.

Although their intent was clearly to teach spiritual truths and to promote direct and ecstatic communion with Allah, their theology also left room for the physical act of lovemaking.

Muhyiddin Ibn 'Arabi (1165–1240 CE) was a poet, teacher, philosopher, and mystic whose writings focus on everything from the spiritual wisdom of the prophets to metaphysics, cosmology, psychology, and jurisprudence. He also wrote poetry that is clearly based on an actual love relationship.

His collection of love poems called *Tarjuman al-ashwaq* (The Interpreter of Yearnings) was inspired by a young woman named Nizam, whom he met during his first pilgrimage to Mecca. These poems are so erotically charged that he was forced, or felt compelled, to write a long commentary explaining how they actually deal with spiritual truths and not Nizam's charms, as one critic accused.

Although the Sufi mystics may not have articulated a direct metaphysical link between human sexual activity and the divine, as the Kabbalah and the *Zohar* seem to do, they certainly weren't shy about using erotic poetic imagery to convey their understanding of the divine or to critique ideas about God that they believed were too small. Just consider this poem by Hafiz (c. 1320–1389 CE).

Tiny Gods

Some gods say, the tiny ones,
"I am not here in your vibrant, moist lips
That need to beach themselves upon
The golden shore of a
Naked body."

Some gods say, "I am not
The scarred yearning in the unrequited soul;
I am not the blushing cheek
Of every star and
Planet –

I am not the applauding Chef
Of those precious secretions that can distill
The whole mind into a perfect wincing jewel, if only
For a moment;
Nor do I reside in every pile of sweet warm dung
Born of earth's
Gratuity."

Some gods say, the ones we need to hang,
"Your mouth is not designed to know His,
Love was not born to consume
The luminous Realms."

Dear ones,
Beware of the tiny gods frightened men
Create
To bring an anesthetic relief
To their sad
Days.[17]

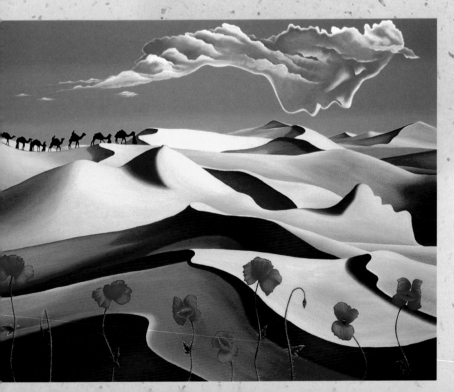

Perhaps it is this awareness of the vastness and beauty of God, and this ability to experience God in everything, especially every form of human love, that makes these ancient spiritual masters so popular today.

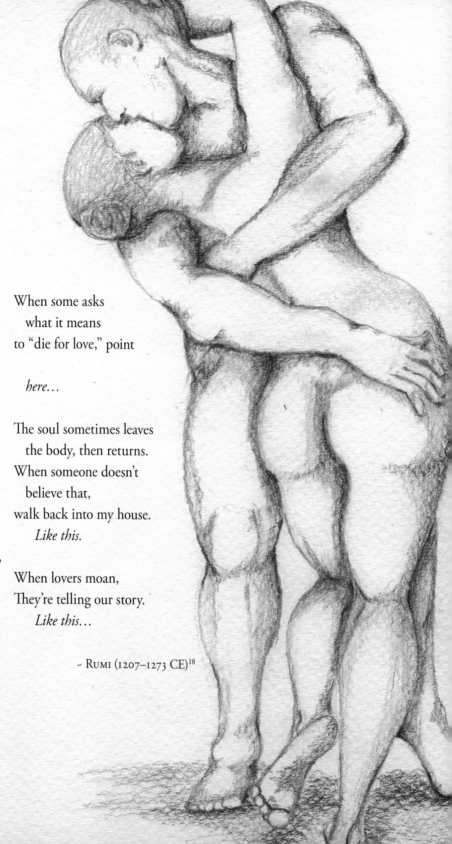

Like This

If anyone asks you
how the perfect satisfaction
of all our sexual wanting
will look, lift your face
and say,
    Like this.

When someone mentions the gracefulness
of the nightsky, climb up on the roof
and dance and say,

Like this?

If anyone wants to know what "spirit" is,
or what "God's fragrance" means,
lean your head toward him or her.
Keep your face there close.

    Like this.

When someone quotes the old poetic image
about clouds gradually uncovering the moon,
slowly loosen knot by knot the strings
of your robe.

    Like this?

If anyone wonders how Jesus raised the dead,
don't try to explain the miracle.
Kiss me on the lips.

Like this. Like this.

When some asks
    what it means
to "die for love," point

    here...

The soul sometimes leaves
    the body, then returns.
When someone doesn't
    believe that,
walk back into my house.
    Like this.

When lovers moan,
They're telling our story.
    Like this...

    ~ RUMI (1207–1273 CE)[18]

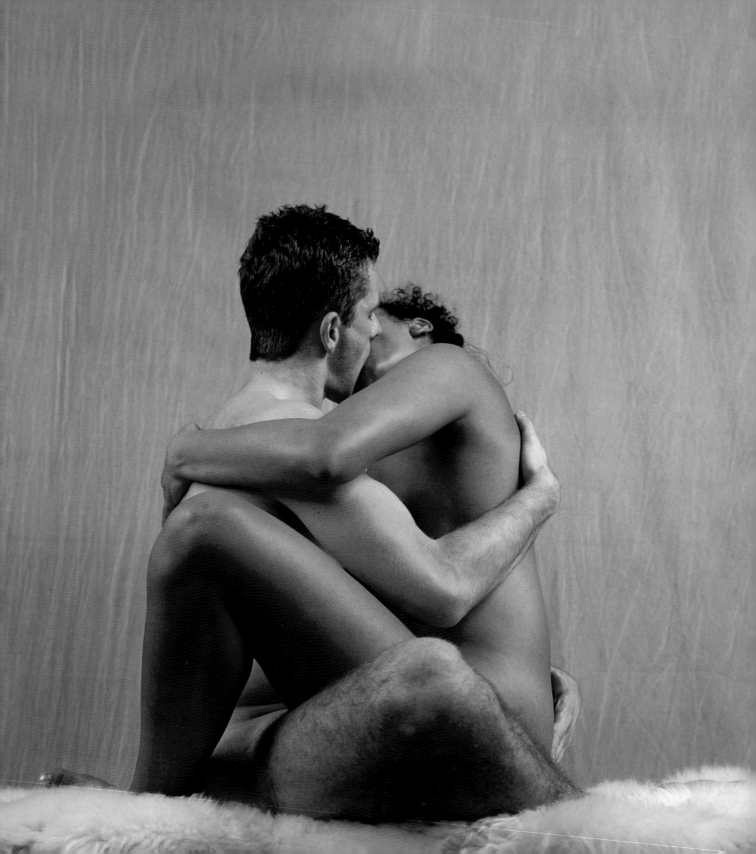

TANTRISM

While the Christian, Jewish, and Sufi love mystics gave voice to the erotic nature of the impulse that drove them to seek union with the divine, none of them embraced the actual sex act as a *spiritual practice* that could bring about mystical union. This possibility is the contribution of the Tantric and Taoist traditions.

It would be difficult to find a sex manual or a book on sacred sexuality today that didn't make at least passing reference to Tantric sex. For those who are truly interested, there are entire books and DVDs devoted exclusively to the topic. Many of these are bought and sold on the premise that the techniques they teach will enhance lovemaking by allowing the man to delay his orgasm, or by enabling him to have multiple orgasms without ejaculating, or by increasing the number and intensity of the woman's orgasms.

In other words, the enjoyment of orgasm or the improvement of some aspect of the sensual experience or the couple's relationship is often the implied or stated goal. While there is nothing wrong with this per se, the pursuit of pleasure as an end in itself was not part of the original Tantric tradition. This focus on orgasm and pleasure really belongs to Neo-Tantrism.

Tantrism was originally meant to help the individual achieve the spiritual goal of "liberation (*mukti*)…understood as transcendence of the ego personality," or ordinary consciousness. The attainment of this state is usually described as "unexcelled bliss (*ananda*), or delight."[19] The specific sexual techniques taught, if any, and the abilities achieved were merely a path to this destination, not the destination itself.

Tantrism is based on a complex philosophy and has many different schools, both in Hinduism and in Buddhism. Although these schools often contradict each other, there are a few ideas that all Tantric schools hold in common.

One of these ideas is that the divine is not separate from the physical world of creation. This means that the divine is present or manifest in everything, including in each person. It is, in fact, our true nature or condition.

Moreover, all schools of Tantrism view the divine as comprising both feminine and masculine principles. In Hindu Tantrism, these principles are called *Shakti* and *Shiva*, respectively. *Shakti*, the feminine principle, is the dynamic aspect of the divine, and represents creation, matter, nature, and change. *Shiva*, the male principle, is the static aspect of the divine, and represents absolute awareness or consciousness.

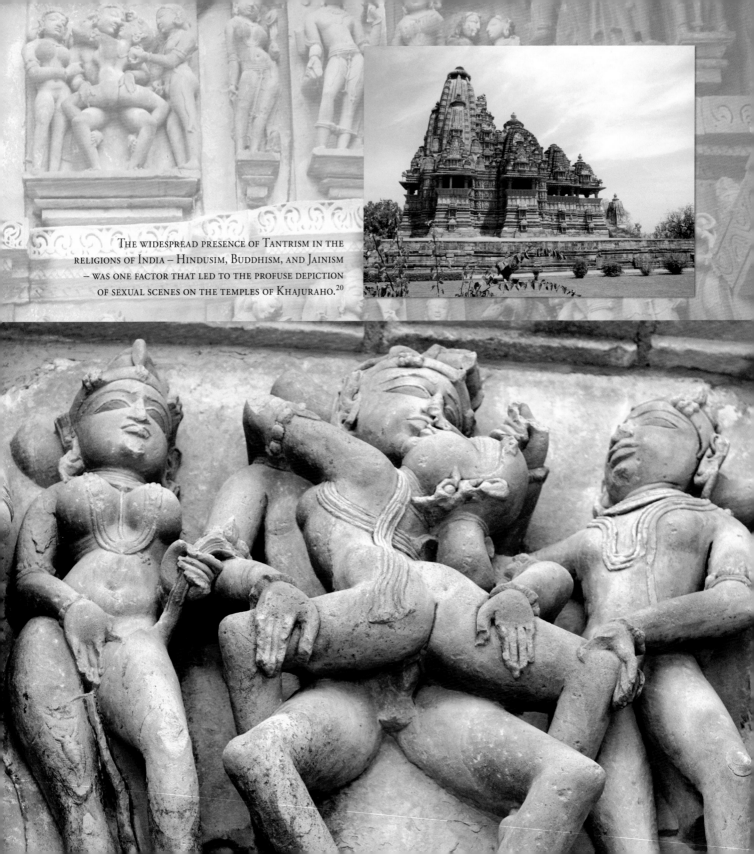

THE WIDESPREAD PRESENCE OF TANTRISM IN THE RELIGIONS OF INDIA – HINDUSIM, BUDDHISM, AND JAINISM – WAS ONE FACTOR THAT LED TO THE PROFUSE DEPICTION OF SEXUAL SCENES ON THE TEMPLES OF KHAJURAHO.[20]

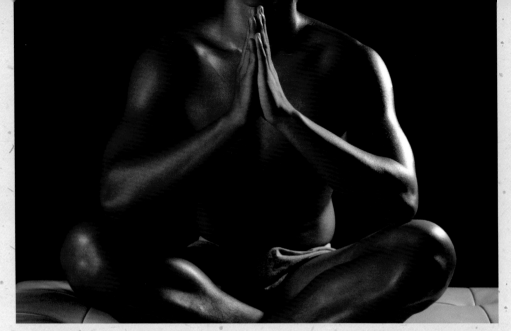

On the highest level of existence, Shakti and Shiva (personified as Goddess and God), exist in a state of inseparable wholeness. Their love-play (*lila*) is what creates the universe.

In simple terms, the goal of the Tantric practitioner is to recapture this transcendent wholeness or balance, this union of Shiva and Shakti, within him- or herself.

Exactly how this is done varies between Tantric schools, but there are two main approaches: right-hand Tantrism and left-hand Tantrism.

Right-hand Tantrism is similar to medieval Christian, Jewish, and Sufi love mysticism in that the core ritual of sexual union is not taken literally, but is understood in a purely symbolic or allegorical way. The union of male and female happens within the individual psyche – which, like the divine, is polarized into masculine and feminine. This union is the culmination of meditation and yogic practices, such as kundalini yoga, which is designed to awaken kundalini or Shakti (feminine principle) energy. This energy travels up from the lowest chakra to the crown chakra, the seat of Shiva (the male principle), thus reuniting the two.

In left-hand Tantrism, the core ritual of sexual union, called *maithuna*, is taken literally. This highly ritualized form of intercourse is the fifth and final element of a much longer ceremony, and represents an enactment of the fusion between Shiva and Shakti. As in the *hieros gamos* ritual of the Goddess traditions, the participants understand themselves to be incarnations of the God and Goddess in that moment.

Taoism

The Taoist approach to sacred sexuality shares many things in common with Tantrism. First and foremost is the notion that the realm of the *tao*, or the "Way," is characterized by a balance or harmony between the feminine and the masculine, between the *yin* and *yang*, respectively. This balance or harmony can be described as *dynamic* because although the *tao* is utterly still, it is nevertheless the source of all movement and creation. This perfectly balanced movement is beautifully illustrated in the familiar *t'ai ch'i* or *yin-yang* symbol.

Like the Tantric gurus, the Taoist masters were experts at controlling and directing the life force or life energy of the body, which they called *ch'i* (or *prana* in Tantrism).

Where the Tantric and Taoist masters differ is in the goal each sought. The Tantric masters wanted to transcend the body-mind, whereas the Taoist masters were primarily concerned with accumulating psychosexual energy, which they used to rejuvenate the body. Also, whereas the *maithuna* ceremony of left-hand Tantrism was a very solemn and ritualized form of intercourse, the Taoists encouraged variety and playfulness.

The union of man and woman is like the mating of Heaven and Earth. It is because of their correct mating that Heaven and Earth last forever. Humans have lost this secret and have therefore become mortal. By knowing it the Path to Immortality is opened.

- Shang-ku-san-ti
(Ancient Taoist Text)

EMBRACING THE BODY

At the beginning of the chapter, I said I found it liberating to learn how other religious traditions have understood the relationship between sex and the divine. I especially appreciate that most of these ancient traditions, though not all, understand that we do not have to leave our bodies behind in our search for God and, more importantly perhaps, a spiritual way of *being*.

As Georg Feuerstein says, "The Kingdom of God is near... We do not have to go anywhere – especially not up – to open that hidden portal; rather we must be willing to be fully present *in* and as *our* body."[21]

To say it another way, the spirituality that appeals to me is about *incarnation*. It is about recognizing and accepting that the body is the home or temple of the spirit, and the vehicle through which spirit expresses itself in the physical world. Transcendent experiences may come, but, in one of the many paradoxes of the spiritual life, I do not have to ignore my body or necessarily repress or redirect its desires in order to experience them. Rather, an incarnational spirituality invites me to live in the world of the senses, and to find God there.

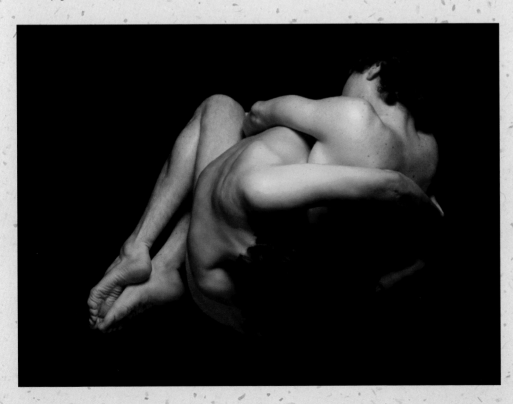

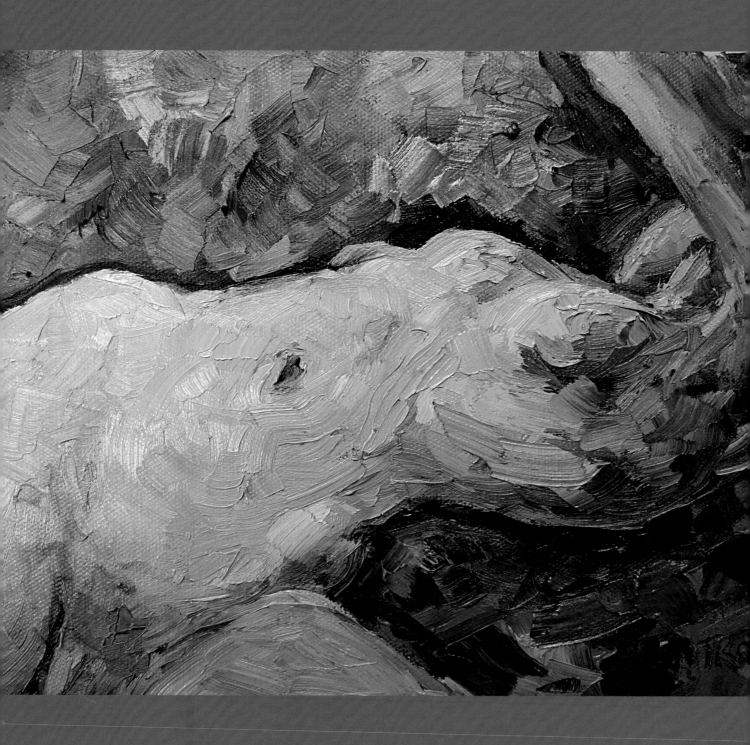

3
Sacred Female Sexuality

LOIS HUEY-HECK

*Collectively we have not quite known
what to do with… the power of sexuality – its potential
for new life, for passion, for destruction, for joy,
for religious experience…*

~ GERTRUDE MUELLER NELSON

Early in the 21st century, female sexuality and female spirituality remain two highly charged subjects and are among the most confused areas of our collective lives, according to author and ethicist Mary Pellauer. I could hardly agree more. Sexual-spirituality and spiritual-sexuality carry the potential of great blessing and great wounding – two sides of a numinous power.

The greatest challenge for me during the writing of this chapter has been to enter wholeheartedly into a celebration of sacred feminine sexuality while not denying the brokenness in and around us. Even as we approach the celebrative side of female sexuality, I never want to forget those who suffer due to destructive manifestations of sex.

Confronted with this reality during the research for this chapter, I was dropped into an unexpected grief so pervasive that it stopped me in my tracks and ultimately caused me to surrender into a chrysalis-like state. The cocoon that wound around those immobilized weeks was layered with strands of personal story, threads of experience from the sisterhood, and braided filaments of pain, "righteous" anger, despair, resolve, and mystical hope.

Memories surfaced of times when I knew myself to be part of the larger web of life. One of the most significant of these was when my newborn child was placed *on* my body for the first time. I was flooded with euphoria and gratitude (not to mention relief) for the miracle of life. Yet even as those tears of joy were still wet on my cheeks, I was seized with sorrow for all my sisters who carry a baby and endure the rigours of birth only to lose their precious child. In that moment, I felt the sisterhood of women in my bones and blood like never before. I was touched by the truth of women's experience within the facts of birth, life, and death – the ways our bodies and sexuality themselves are our gateways into and connections with the Absolute.

During this chosen immersion into sacred female sexuality, my life has been melted down once again. But oh, the glimpses of glory – the push and pull, the stretching of wings towards flight!

The image on this page is by Maria Sibylla Merian, the artist-naturalist who first discovered the miracle that is metamorphosis. Around 1700, she and a daughter lived in Suriname for two years, studying and painting the entire life cycle of many insects and the plants they lived on. Three hundred years later, while I was researching for this chapter, this particular painting showed up in a pile of magazine clippings. This image, *Branch of Pomegranate and Split Fruit,* bridges the metaphor of metamorphosis with our look into the blossom that is female spiritual-sexuality.

When this chapter itself was in the unformed chrysalis stage, as I wondered what "shape" it was going to assume, Spirit guidance came to me: "It's to be a…flower." And literally brushstroke-by-brushstroke, line-by-line, thought-by-thought, this chapter took the form of a flower – a triune blossom with three full-coloured voluptuous outer petals, three soft and sensuous centre petals, and a hint of the potential to bear fruit.

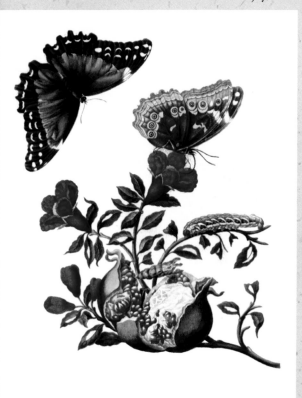

To See a World in a
Grain of Sand
And a Heaven
in a Wild Flower,
Hold Infinity in
the palm of your hand
And Eternity in an hour.
- WILLIAM BLAKE

Three Full-Coloured Voluptuous Outer Petals

The outer petals of a blossom are usually the first thing we notice. We love their colours and exotic shapes. Being that they are the sex organs of the plant, attractive blossoms are just doing their job.

We're going to look at the sacredness of female sexuality by considering first the three large outer petals of the flower – the petals that symbolize *who we are* as sexual-spiritual women: *body* (presence and our sacred physical-sexual selves), *mind* (integration of our spiritual psychology/beliefs), and *feelings* (relationship as outcome of our inner marriage of masculine and feminine).

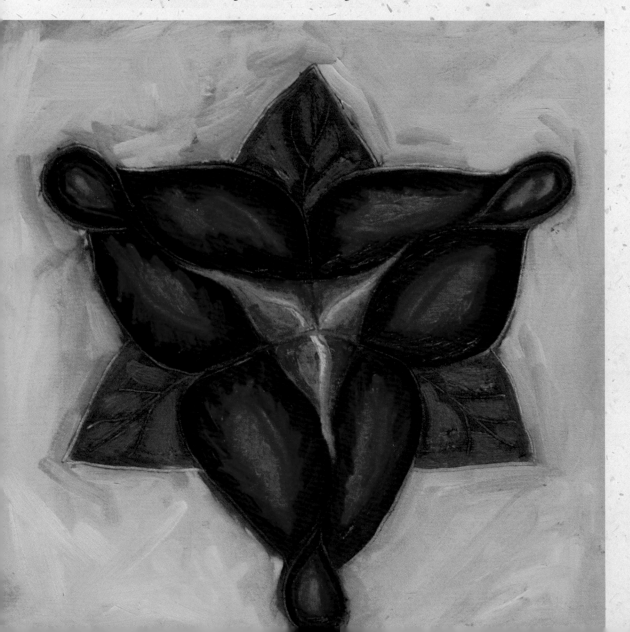

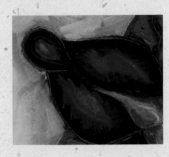

If, to paraphrase Woody Allen, life is eighty percent about showing up, then we need to bring as much of the fullness of ourselves as possible into every moment, every encounter. This is nowhere more true than when it comes to spiritually conscious sexuality. While it's true that a good portion of sex happens "between the ears" in the form of thoughts, ideas, and dearly held beliefs, sexual expression has a whole lot to do with our physical, material selves – our bodies.

I remember hearing the story of a wise person who said it was his goal to live fully in his body before he died. I didn't get it at the time, but I understand it better now – now that I've noticed how much of my life I spend dwelling in the past and future, now that I've seen how often I live from the neck up, now that I've noticed how easily my attention wanders from the present moment, and now that I know how persistent my negative body image is. Slowly I am beginning to comprehend how it can be that we touch eternity not in some grandiose abstraction, but by being present as fully as possible in each moment. Now, as it turns out, is the point of communion between the material-temporal and the spiritual-eternal.

The most precious gift we can offer others is our presence. When mindfulness embraces those we love, they will bloom like flowers.

~ THICH NHAT HANH

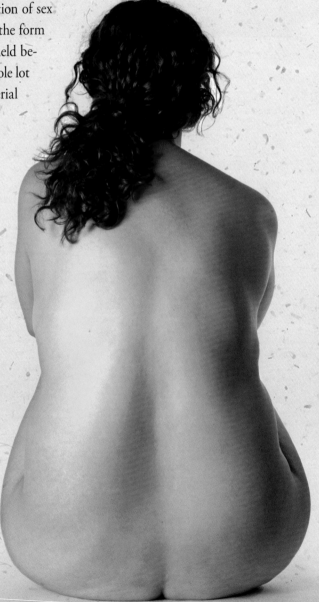

Today we still have a love-hate relationship with our sexuality — we are obsessed with sexuality, self-gratification, and the body on the one hand and we fear and loath them on the other. Surveys reveal that a majority of girls and women struggle with negative body image. Having grown up dissatisfied with the appearance and behaviour of our bodies, it often takes practice to learn how to occupy our miraculous bodies consciously, consistently, and gratefully. Mature acceptance of the bodies we have helps us inhabit them more fully and joyfully, deepening the experience of sacred sexuality.

The pages that follow are an appreciation of the female genitalia in word and image. The first of the voluptuous outer petals is embodiment and presence. Like velvet to the touch…

Knowing and using correct language for our genitals helps affirm a healthy sexuality. Knowing some of the respectful and sacred language for genitals and sexuality can further enrich our experience. This is not to say that other kinds of language shouldn't be used in our pillow talk — but it is to affirm the value of a full and mature vocabulary. The words and images we use do reflect our attitudes and beliefs, and inform them in return.

Language is obviously not the only issue around our bodies and our sacred sexuality, but it is one place we can make immediate and tangible changes that can help us accept and appreciate the miracle that every body is. The opportunity before us is to "make way" in our bodies, minds, and emotions for the reunion of our earthy, moist sexuality with our ethereal, fiery spirituality.

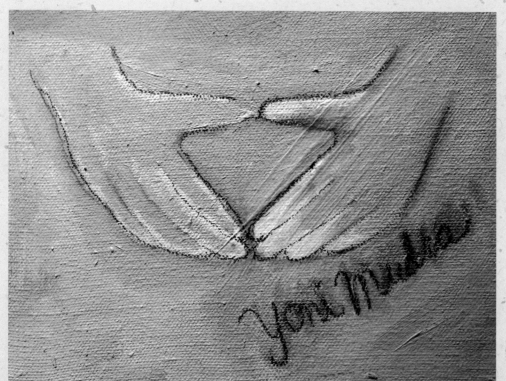

The word yoni *neither carries any of the linguistic undercurrents of clinical detachment of words such as vulva or vagina nor has any of the pornographic, immature, and often derogatory connotations of words like cunt and similar expressions.*

— *The Encyclopedia of Erotic Wisdom*

67

Vulva
The Lover's View

The Latin/medical term vulva *refers to the outer and visible parts of the female genital system, also called the pudenda, that surrounds the opening to the vagina.*

– THE ENCYCLOPEDIA OF EROTIC WISDOM

This painterly view of the vulva is obviously not the casual view one may see in a public change room. This is an up-close and intimate view – the lover's view. It's more a visual poem than a photograph, and while it's essentially accurate it takes some obvious license with colour and shape, and offers a more open view – the view a lover might see.

Vulva: the primary Tantric object of worship, symbolized variously by a triangle, fish, double-pointed oval, horseshoe, egg, fruits, etc. Personifying the yoni, the Goddess Kali bore the title of Cunti or Kunda, root of the ubiquitous Indo-European word "cunt" and all its relatives: cunnus, cunte, cunning, cunctipotent, ken, kin, and country.

– BARBARA WALKER

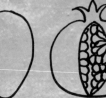

Pubis
The triangle of hair which covers the mons veneris and most of the labia majora.

Mons Pubis/Veneris (pubic mound)
This cushion of tissue protects the pubic bone and separates into the labia majora.
>> Also known as *the Mound of Venus.*

Prepuce (hood of clitoris)
The fold of skin that covers the shaft of the clitoris forms a protective hood over the tip of the clitoris.

Labia Majora (outer lips)
These outer lips start at the mons veneris and end at the perineum. The outer protective folds are covered with pubic hair while the inside is smooth and hairless. They often swell during arousal.

Labia Minora (inner lips)
The smaller lips are smooth skin in various shades of pink. They contain glands that moisten the sensitive tissues and also may swell and change colour during arousal.
>> Also known as *the nymphae.*

Vestibule
The entrance chamber to the vagina is the area enclosed by the labia minora. It contains the openings of the urethra and vagina, the vulvovaginal glands, erectile tissue, and mucous glands.

Hymen
A membranous fold of skin may partially cover the opening to the vagina.

Pelvic Floor Muscles
Commonly known as the love muscles, this group of muscles can be trained and used to increase sexual pleasure.

Glans Clitoridus (tip)

This is the smallest and the only visible part of the clitoris. Containing a large number of nerve endings, it's highly sensitive. During sexual arousal, it can enlarge and change colour.

>> Also known as *the Lowndes Crown, pearl, clit, and clitoral crown.*

Urethral Orifice (urinary opening)

The urethra is the tube by which urine moves from the bladder out of the body.

Vaginal Glans

This small area below the clitoral crown and above the opening to the vagina is highly sensitive and flexible, moving in and out of the vagina during intercourse.

Vaginal Orifice (opening to vagina)

This is the entry to the muscular tube that leads from the vestibule to the cervix and uterus. The walls of the vagina gently fold in and touch each other when not dilated. The vagina itself is not visible unless dilated. It is a pocket of smooth, soft, pink skin.

Orifice of Vulvovaginal Glands

Located near the lower labia minora, these two glands secrete a thick protein into the vestibule, apparently to provide a stimulating sexual odor.

>> Also known as the *vestibular glands or Bartholin's glands.*

Perineum

The area between the vulva and anus is involved with the muscles of the pelvic floor and is sensitive to contact. >> Often mentioned in *Taoist and Tantric texts.*

Perineal Sponge

Located beneath the perineum, this is sensitive tissue that fills with blood during sexual arousal.

The Yoni Yantra or triangle was known as the Primordial Image, representing the Great Mother as a source of all life. As the genital focus of her divine energy, the Yantra was adored as a geometrical symbol, as the cross was adored by Christians. The ceremony of baptismal rebirth often involved being pulled through a giant yoni. Those who underwent this ceremony were styled "Twice-born."

— Barbara Walker, *The Woman's Encyclopedia of Myths and Secrets*

In his book on Northwest Coast art, anthropologist Wilson Duff wrote that he described the "male" forms as phallic (when suggestive of a penis) and phalliform (when they're illustrative of same) and went on to say, "What we do not seem to have recognized until now is that the opposite is equally true. While it presents a more difficult problem of depiction, [some] of the images can be said to be "vulviform" and many more just "vulvic."

Mary Carlson of Harvard Medical School has coined the term "liberation biology" to describe the use of biological insights to heal our psychic wounds, understand our fears, and make the most of what we have and of those who will have us and love us. …What better place to begin the insurrection than at the doors to the palace we've lived in all these years?

— Natalie Angier, *Woman: An Intimate Geography*

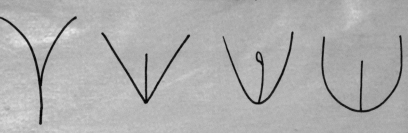

Clitoris

The clitoris is the only known organ of either the female or the male body that exists solely for pleasure.

Most of the clitoris is hidden from view with only its tip (also known as the glans or crown) visible. It's a relatively large structure of erectile tissue with three primary parts.

THE WHOLE CLITORIS

❶ Crura (medical term meaning legs)
A fork with two crura runs downward and inward below the clitoral bulbs at their respective sides of the outer lips.

❷ Crown (head/tip/glans)
Often referred to as the clitoris, it is actually the smallest part of the whole clitoris and the only visible part. It contains a large number of nerve endings, making it highly sensitive. During sexual arousal, it can enlarge and also may change colour.

❸ Shaft
The shaft becomes erect and enlarged (as does the crown) by the increased blood pressure that occurs during sexual stimulation. It's highly sensitive and moves involuntarily when touched.
>> Also known as *the corpus*.

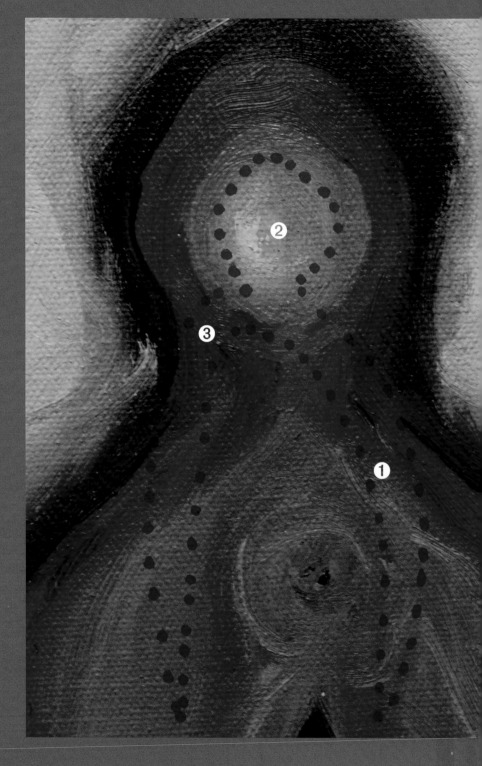

From the Greek *kleitoris*, "divine, famous, goddess-like." Greek myth personified the phallus as priapus and the clitoris as an Amazon queen named Kleite, ancestral mother of the Kleitae, a tribe of warrior women who founded a city in Italy. In Corinth, Kleite was a princess "whom Artemis made grow tall and strong," an allegory of her erection.

~ Barbara Walker

Penis Envy. P'shaw…
I have two words to put an end to that kind of foolish thinking, multiple orgasms.
…I guarantee the genital envy table will be turned for good.

~ Karen Salmonsohn,
The Clitourist

I see our culture's common practice of mislabeling female genitalia as a serious matter indeed. It is true that [North] Americans do not surgically remove the clitoris and the labia, as is practiced on countless girls and women in other cultures. Instead we do the job linguistically – a psychic genital mutilation, if you will. Language can be as powerful and swift as the surgeon's knife. What is not named does not exist.

~ Harriet Goldhor Lerner

Vagina

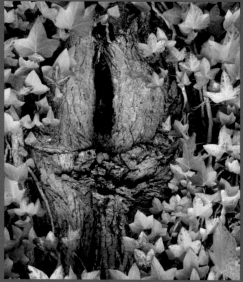

IRONICALLY, THE FEMALE GENITALS THAT WE CAN SEE ARE OFTEN MISTAKENLY REFERRED TO AS THE VAGINA, ONE OF THE VERY PARTS WE CAN'T SEE.

Vagina: A deeply folded, elastic, and muscular tube the vagina connects the vestibule to the cervix. The vagina is highly lubricated by its mucous membranes and plays, in concert with the vaginal muscles, a most important role in sexual union, a role often neglected in medical textbooks. Of course, it also constitutes the pathway that must be travelled by the menstrual fluid, by the sperm cells on their way to the ovum, and, at birth, by the newborn human. The discussion over whether or not there are vaginal and/or clitoral and/or G-spot orgasms is still not concluded, yet it anyway becomes superfluous when we consider the Yoni* as a holistic system.

~ *The Encyclopedia of Erotic Wisdom*

*Yoni is Sanskrit term meaning "womb," "origin," and "source" and refers to the female pubic region.

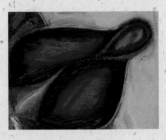

On the desk beside my computer sits the image *Esther, Cassandra and Me*. The central figure working at the drawing table is me. On my left, the somewhat wan Esther stands stiffly, watching. Sitting cross-legged on the right side of the drawing table and facing straight forward is the full-bodied Cassandra. *Esther, Cassandra and Me* is a family photo of sorts; it records a group of relationships in my inner world.

Although we don't always like to admit it, we all have an inner family or community of some sort. They're a fact of life whether we're closely connected, estranged, indifferent, or anywhere along that continuum. Even though we don't always *consciously* think of these parts of ourselves, we know *of them* through the conversations that go on in our heads, and through statements such as "One part of me wants to go, an-

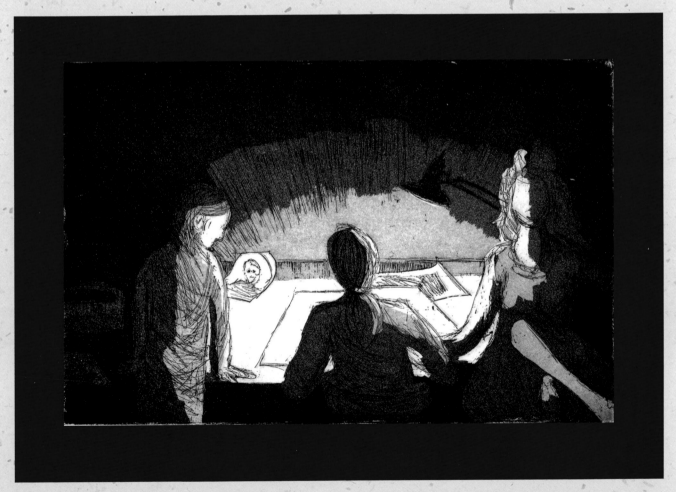

ESTHER, CASSANDRA AND ME BY LOIS HUEY-HECK

other part wants to stay, and another part wishes…" or "On the one hand, I think we should… on the other hand, I feel strongly that we shouldn't."

For most of us, the fact that there are several parts to our personalities should be no cause for alarm. On the contrary – the members of our inner families exist to serve the greater good of our lives, even though, just as with outer family members, it doesn't always appear that way!

Esther and Cassandra represent *within me* something pervasive in our culture, which is known as the Mary-Eve, Madonna-Harlot, or the virgin-whore split. Jungian analyst and author Marion Woodman observes this cultural epidemic as one of separating our love from our lust. Sadly, although not surprisingly, women and girls – steeped in long-standing traditions – have internalized the belief that our sexuality is sinful, dirty, and dangerous. This affects us personally and it affects our relationships.

Esther, Cassandra and I were just meeting at the time I drew us. They held each other in utter disdain and I didn't like either of them very much. I was embarrassed by old-fashioned Esther's dry, wizened nervousness. I resented the way the femme-fatale-wanna-be Cassandra broke out of my control, lusting after "inappropriate" men and, well, *lusting* period.

Reconciliation starts so humbly… "Hello, Esther; I'm glad to meet you at last. I'm sorry I haven't really seen you before. I want to thank you for all the ways you have worked to keep me safe from the compulsive part of my sexual desire; I know it hasn't always been easy. I also realize that I haven't always appreciated you and your efforts and I hope you will accept my sincere apology." And "Hi, Cassandra; we need to talk. We're tripping over each other and I realize that I need to hear what you want, what you yearn for. And I need to tell you what I need…"

To be spiritual means essentially to take responsibility for our inner journey…

– Wayne Teasdale,
The Mystic Heart

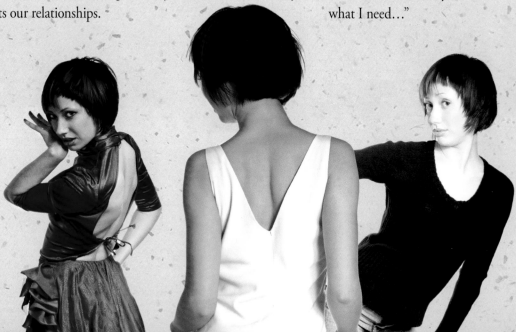

Once conversations like this begin we *must* be prepared to listen to the responses. They may come in word-thought, bodily sensation, emotion, image, or a combination of these. Esther and Cassandra have had some things to say to me over the years that haven't always been easy to hear. But intentional "meetings" like this are one of the most effective ways I've found to heal inner rifts and continue the journey to wholeness. Jung gave these truthful inner conversations a name. He called them "active imagination."

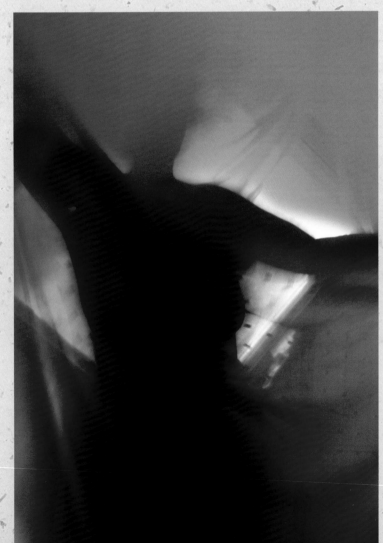

I've been mindfully relating to Cassandra and Esther for over two decades now, and in my mind, journal, and sketchbook the conversations continue. These days, Esther and Cassandra are great friends. Together we are practicing being "juicy" within the relative safety of a long-term life partnership. Cassandra doesn't have to act out in ways that could hurt me or someone else, so Esther has lightened up. We all laugh more, play more, and take more chances sexually and spiritually – all the while tending the outer relationship, keeping the home fires burning, and seeking ways to offer service to the world. Our three-way relationship has virtually eliminated the split between my love and my lust. The chaste and spiritual Esther is sexier and more spontaneous, the libidinous and earthy Cassandra is more reverent, and we're all wiser.

We are all sexual in our DNA, our cells and bones. And no matter whether we are on a life-path of celibacy, in a time of abstinence (chosen or circumstantial), or sexually active – our sexuality is a fact of life. And because, as Carl Jung said, "What we don't live consciously comes to us as fate," it's much better for us to befriend our spirituality and our sexuality and introduce them to each other. Our spirituality benefits greatly from being centred and grounded (a body is particularly good for that), and our sexuality becomes ecstatic when integrated with Spirit.

Carl Jung understood the integration of parts of our personalities (e.g., our sexual "Eve" and spiritual "Mary") to be our "apprentice-piece" for the creation of a deep relationship between inner masculine and feminine – what he called our "masterpiece." Marion Woodman speaks of it as well (emphasis mine).

> Relationship, as I understand it, has to do with the exquisitely tuned harmonics between two people who are attempting to become conscious of their personal psychology. The mystery of each individual is holy, and the mystery which brings each into relationship with the other is tenuous, invisible and sacred… For such a relationship to exist, the partners must be constantly responsive to the ever finer tuning of the *maturing masculine and feminine* both in themselves and in the other.[1]

Woodman says that the *inner marriage* of masculine and feminine is our greatest creative act. She explains why this matters to our spiritual-sexual lives by adding, "The inner marriage is what makes the *outer* marriage [or union] possible."[2]

Before we can consider inner engagement – let alone inner marriage – we need to acknowledge that we are both feminine

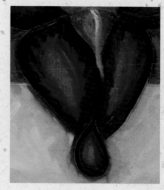

and masculine. This takes some relationship savvy, because the inner masculine for a woman – called the animus – is more elusive than other parts of ourselves. We can start "dating" by introducing ourselves and having some meaningful conversations (inner dialogue). "Courting" escalates as we develop a relationship of respect and trust, and continue to nurture it. The establishment of a mutually respectful, ongoing, and intimate relationship with the animus consummates the inner marriage.

"Right relationship" with the animus means that as women we're empowered to bring our feminine creativity (e.g., work, art, religious impulse, acts of service, family-making) into being in the world. We don't have to become "iron maidens" – overload-

In a woman the animus is the masculine energy and the inner feminine is the woman's own female-soul.

– MARION WOODMAN

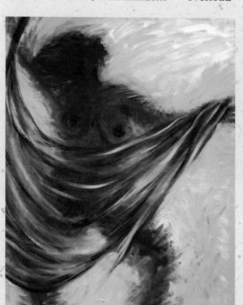

When the masculine is unbound, and the feminine is unveiled, then together they interact within and without.

– MARION WOODMAN

75

Projection in itself is neither good nor bad; it is what we do with it that counts.

~ JOHN A. SANFORD

ed with masculine energy, fighting our way into old power structures. Nor need we be retiring wallflowers unable to live our own destinies (like the "good woman" behind every successful man). Animus energy *needs* to be doing, wants to be seen, and yearns to illuminate and give form and expression to the feminine principle. It's meant to be a symbiotic relationship.

There is another reason to nurture a relationship with our inner masculine. There's a particular quality to the animus that can cause unexpected turbulence in our lives.

When we don't relate to our inner maleness consciously, we may find it inadvertently attaching itself to someone else. This phenomenon is known as projection.

If we look back at our lives, most of us will find memories of strong or unlikely attractions. These attractions, or projections, are as unpredictable as they are intense. The early stages of animus attraction can be so heady and electric that it's easy to believe we've found our soul mate. But while some of our projections *do* lead us into long-term relationships that grow into genuine love, we shouldn't necessarily jump into bed with the objects of our desire.

Once I had such a strong experience of projection that I didn't know what hit me. I was walking along talking to a man I hardly knew and was struck by a lightning-bolt of sexual attraction. I hadn't seen it coming. I was happily married to someone else. Having never before been blindsided by such a strong and inappropriate sexual attraction, I mistakenly took it too literally at first and felt immense guilt for these feelings. Fortunately, I had done some deep inner work and my love-relationship mattered deeply to me. I did not act on the attraction.

I'd *like* to tell you that it was just that simple. The truth is that the force of the attraction stirred up my inner and outer worlds in some uncomfortable ways, and there were times of white-knuckled resistance to my aroused feelings. In time, by grace, and with as much consciousness as I could muster, I came to understand something of the mysterious attraction. This outer man appeared to be "everything I was not," which made him a perfect carrier of the unfamiliar parts of myself. In the latter stages of the projection, I came to know that the "qualities" I saw in him were my own qualities.

Through the inner dialogue of active imagination, I began to claim some of my strength and authority in the outer world. Through the process of reflecting on the ex-

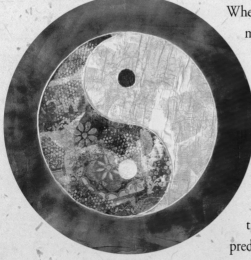

THE QUINTESSENTIAL SYMBOLIC REPRESENTATION OF MALE-FEMALE IN RIGHT RELATIONSHIP IS THE YIN AND YANG SYMBOL OF THE ORIENT. YIN AND YANG ARE PICTURED WITH FLUID BOUNDARIES AND IN EACH THERE IS A "DROP" OF THE OTHER.

76

perience (writing and drawing in my journal), deeper levels of meaning were revealed. In conversations with soul-friends, it was all put into perspective within the larger context of my life, and I was well accompanied as I worked with the "charge" of the animus relationship. Re-claiming these parts of ourselves is called "withdrawing our projections" and it's essential to the health of our outer sexual-spiritual relationships.

By nature, we're never completely clear of all projection. Being conscious of our inner marriage, though, goes a long way towards reducing the frequency and intensity of projections and helps us, when they do occur, to spot them quickly for what they are.

Nurturing an inner marriage is the work of a lifetime and is not a strictly sequential process. These are organic, spiral, floral processes: we work, we discover, we heal… we experience ecstasy, we move on, and we cycle back. All the while remembering that in the economy of Love and Grace nothing is ever lost. John A. Sanford puts it this way:

> Eros needs the enlightenment of a developed consciousness in order to reach its proper goal. Yet without eros, consciousness cannot develop and the goal cannot be reached. In the last analysis, eros is a great mystery. We can talk of sexuality, we can understand projec-

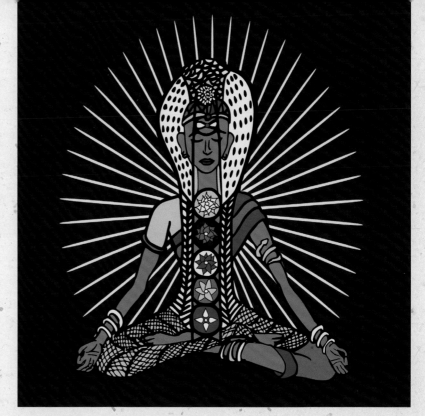

tions…but when we add it all up it comes to zero, for it all ends at the great mystery of Love.[3]

While we have focused here on the inner marriage, it's fair to acknowledge that many events, encounters, and dynamics affect our outer relationships. It's also true that, outside of trauma-recovery work, there's perhaps nothing that affects our sexual relationships more profoundly than the integration of our many selves. The more fully we do this inner work, the richer, more authentic, and more deeply intimate our outer relationships can be.

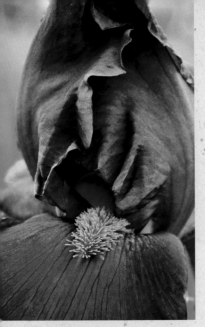

Three Soft and Sensuous Centre Petals: Experience

Have you ever fallen into the soft, seductive centre of an iris and not wanted to come out? It has happened to me more than once. In fact, it's an annual practice of mine in May and June when the large irises are in bloom in our garden. This looking into the gorgeously sexy centres of flowers is my preferred form of voyeurism. The three stories that follow allow us a peek down into the soft, seductive centre of the blossom that is feminine sexual-spiritual experience.

The Colour Purple

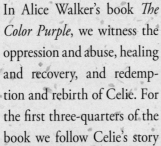
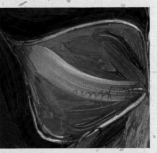

In Alice Walker's book *The Color Purple*, we witness the oppression and abuse, healing and recovery, and redemption and rebirth of Celie. For the first three-quarters of the book we follow Celie's story through her letters to God, but then Celie starts writing to her long-lost sister instead. Celie states emphatically that she has given up on God. She tells her confidant and lover, Shug (short for Sugar), that "the God I been praying and writing to is a man. And act just like all the other mens I know. Trifling, forgitful and lowdown."[4]

Shug is taken aback and tries to budge Celie away from her "blasphemy." For all her wild ways (an overt and sensual sexuality), it turns out that Shug is deeply spiritual. The two women talk about the image of that old white man in the sky and how he doesn't listen to poor coloured women. Shug gets into some beautiful theology as she talks about the God inside each of us (the immanent Divine) and the Holy all around us in trees, birds, wildflowers (the transcendent Divine).

Shug shares the story of how she came to know herself as being connected to everything. She tells Celie of her ecstatic (laughing, crying, running around) response to experiencing the Absolute, the Oneness.

…When it happen, you can't miss it. It sort of like you know what, she say, grinning and rubbing high up on my thigh. *Shug!* I say.

Oh, she say. God love all them feelings. That's some of the best stuff God did. And when you know God loves 'em you enjoys 'em a lot more. You can just relax, go with everything that's going, and praise God by liking what you like.

God don't think it dirty? I ast.

Naw, she say. God made it. Listen, God love everything you love – and a mess of stuff you don't. But more than anything else, God love admiration.

You saying God vain? I ast.

Naw, she say. Not vain, just wanting to share a good thing. I think it pisses God off if you walk by the color purple in a field somewhere and don't notice it.[5]

The conversation continues with Shug talking about how much God loves us, wants to please us, and wants to be loved by us. She instructs Celie on how to find God again by moving beyond the old white man in the sky and seeking God in everyone and everything.

Celie's subsequent letters chronicle the hard process of chasing that old white man out of her prayers. She's often frustrated and thinks it's hopeless; old beliefs die hard. It takes persistent intention over a long time for change and healing to come into Celie's relationship with Life, but that and being well-loved are key ingredients in her metamorphosis.

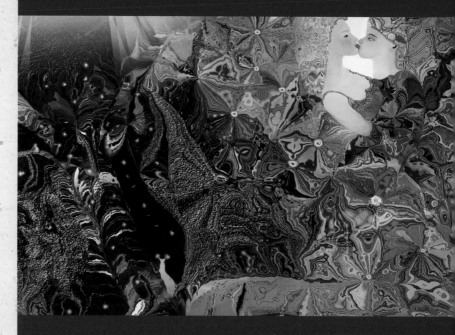

The point of feminine consciousness is not to resolve matter into spirit, or spirit into matter. Rather it is to see spirit in matter and matter in spirit.

~ MARION WOODMAN

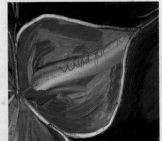

In a compelling essay in *Sexuality and the Sacred*,[6] Mary Pellauer focuses on the moral and ethical implications of female orgasm. In a refreshingly personal and vulnerable act (especially for a scholarly writer), Pellauer shares her own experience of orgasm. Following on Harriet Goldhor Lerner's observation that "what we don't name doesn't exist," I would add that what we do not name in mature, open, and respectful ways is subject to being vulgarized.

Breathing in I calm my body. Breathing out I smile. Dwelling in the present moment, I know this is a wonderful moment!

~ THICH NHAT HANH

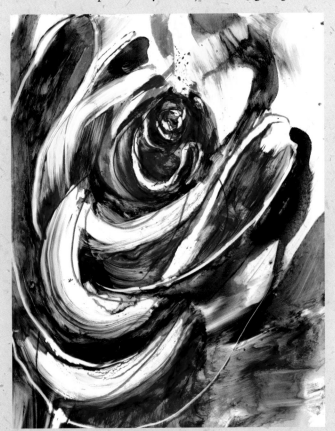

Pellauer names six "elements" in her personal experiences of orgasm: being here and now, varieties of sensations, ecstasy, vulnerability, power, and nothing above can be taken for granted. Her writing for each element is a blend of revelatory stream-of-consciousness, evocative poetry, and unselfconscious reflection – a fine model of deepening into spiritual-sexual maturity. The full text is a great read and I hope this small sample of her first three elements will whet your appetite.

Being Here and Now. Simply stated, this element relates to the practice of being present – easy to say and hard to do with consistency. Most spiritual practices foster the ability to be in the moment – the "eternal now" – the only place where we can meet and be met. I imagine the delight with which Pellauer must have written, "There are no recipes for lovemaking to orgasm (except this one). It is not capable of being routinized." Her main point is that the illusive female orgasm requires faithfulness to what *is* in the moment.

Varieties of Sensations. Pellauer asks, "So, what is it like?" and answers in a poetic style reminiscent of the biblical Song of Songs. Beginning with the skin, she describes the sensate experiences of touch, smell, response, and arousal and evokes for us a delicious encounter. She describes the building of electricity leading to the plateau phase and then to the point of tipping over the edge into orgasm.

If I am lucky, I do go over the edge. Tremors centre in my pelvis, vibrating me like a violin string. As I am shaken from the hips outward my bones turn to lava, languorous liquid fire, heated jelly in the pelvis and thighs, magma coursing down. Sometimes it is not this strong or vibrant… All I can do is remain open to the flaring guidance I receive from the impulses and feelings as they arise…

Pellauer also notices that while the experience is abundantly pleasurable before and during orgasm, orgasm is more for her than just a continuation or deepening of pleasure. There's something else, something more in the experience of orgasm. And that something is…

Ecstasy. "At the moment/eternity of orgasm itself, I melt into existence and it melts into me. I am most fully embodied in this explosion of nerves and also broken open into the cosmos. I am rent open; I am cleaved/joined not only to my partner, but to everything, everything-as-my-beloved (or vice versa), who has also become me."

What follows is a description of how radically Pellauer's sense of herself and her personal boundaries shift – either dissolving away so that she is a part of everything *or* expanding to the point where everything is part of her. She calls this the "quasi-mystical dimension" and shares with us the effect this powerful experience has on her.

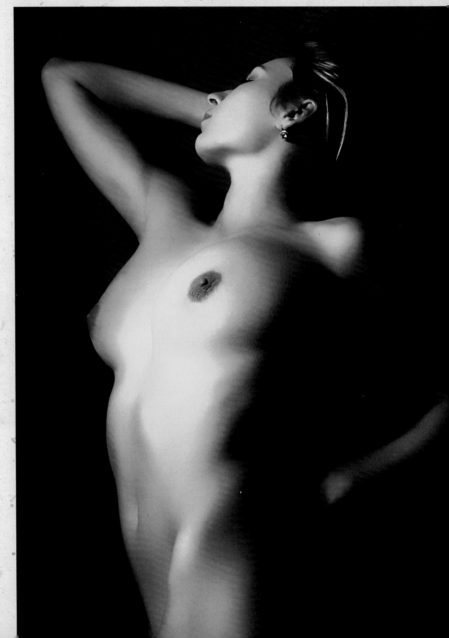

When I am in this state, reverently and greedily cherishing these gracious plains of flesh, whole-self-as-caress, I want to cherish every plane in the world with this same tenderness – the wood of the bedside table, the walls of the room, the grass of the yard outside… all call out to me to caress them in this same tender mood, not to intrude upon them my sexuality, but to cherish them as I cherish our skin-self.

Orgasm is *sui generis* [unique]. It is paradoxical. Ecstasy is what is at stake here. Ek-stasis, standing outside the self, is the closest word for this state. At the same time, it is the most definite incarnation I know outside of childbirth, for in it I am most completely bound to the stimulation of my body. Thus, immanence and transcendence meet here, another paradox.

Orgasm is a gift I receive *from my own body*. My very flesh has this capacity to burst me open to existence, to melt me down into a state in which my connections to the rest of the universe are not only felt, but felt as extremely pleasurable, as joyous.

Let the people say, Amen, Blessed Be, or Namaste…

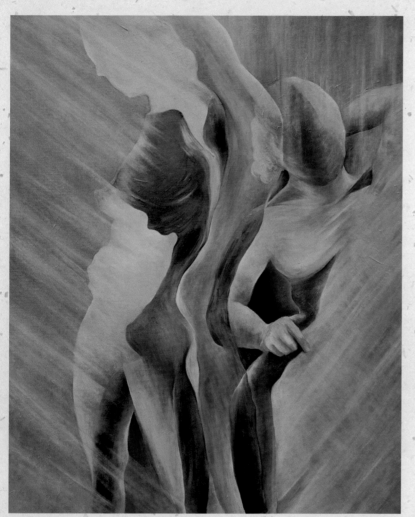

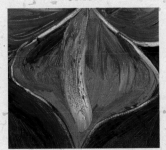

Bright, clear, and cold, it was an early December Saturday morning. At midday I would leave the retreat centre – my soul-home – to head back to my physical- and heart-home where Jim would be waiting. These were the last hours of my four-day silent retreat and the completion of my spiritual direction training. It had been a transformative time and every day had been profound in some way.

The day before leaving, I'd had an experience of such immense Grace that I thought the retreat was over except the leave-taking. My journal for the last morning reads,

8:30 AM… A few more hours here. A concentrated 30 minutes will load the van and clean my room. Holy One – within and beyond – how shall we best spend the next few hours? I wish to enter Silence again here – in this room now? I'd also like to paint some more, walk the labyrinth once again and say goodbye to the lake.

I had it pretty well figured out all right, a fitting wrap-up to four amazing days. But "Life" as John Lennon said "is what happens when we're busy making other plans." My next journal entry reads,

Now it's 10:00 AM. After my last writing I felt called to enter Silence, so I bundled up in my quilt with that organic pomegranate on my lap. I experienced a gold and red pulsing presence – head – heart – gut. Felt huge energy from that pomegranate in my root [energy centre at the base of the spine] and encouraged it up my body above the top of my head [crown]. This is the "place" from which I am to meet the world it seems – even if I can't maintain the intensity – this is the place, this is the state. After a while I got sleepy and laid down to nap which I think I did.

When I "woke" something… happened. Something happened that I have no idea how to write about. Should I write it at all? Will it be diminished if I do – or lost if I don't? What do I *want* to do? I want to start by writing…

Knowing I am a beneficiary of your grace, make me a benefactor to others in your name and by your spirit.

– FROM A TRADITIONAL PRAYER

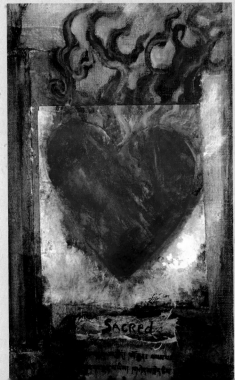

SACRED

I am…

impregnated.

Deliciously,

Advently

Ecstatically

Thoroughly

Impregnated.

It *is* and it *was* sexual and spiritual.
Oh my… God.

Union
and penetration
Surrender
and participation.

Ecstatic/sexual union with the
Beloved. Beloved Wisdom.
Highly feminine *and* highly
masculine. Charged.

It was to be… not split… but…
parted. Opened.
Permeated and filled.
Filled with the sweet red juice of life.

A huge pomegranate uterus. Almost
burning hot juicy.
Burning away the sexual hurts.
Burning away shame.
Burning away vestiges of feeling
unfulfilled.

So erotic-ecstatic that I was sometimes
almost shy –
body writhing, undulating, stretching,
receiving… *feeling!*
Active absorbing vessel.

Why not with the Divine Lover if
with the earthly lover? Why not?

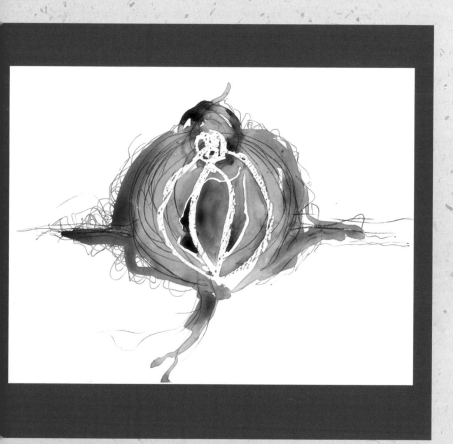

All the lost parts of me… come…
Be a part of this ecstasy.
Every age, every role… come and be
in this ecstatic pleasure.
This joy. This healing.
This redemption. This.

Holy Arousal
Orgasmic but not orgasm. Deeply,
   satisfying.

Desire to explode into an orgasm of
creativity.
Images… such images of
Pomegranate women… juicy redness
(some religious folks will struggle!)

Here I was thinking I was done here
there couldn't possible be more and
then
and *then*

Sexual-spiritual union.

I'm breathless… astounded.
And what (pray tell) does one do after
making love with the Beloved?
Write. Paint…   Shower

And return home open-hearted.

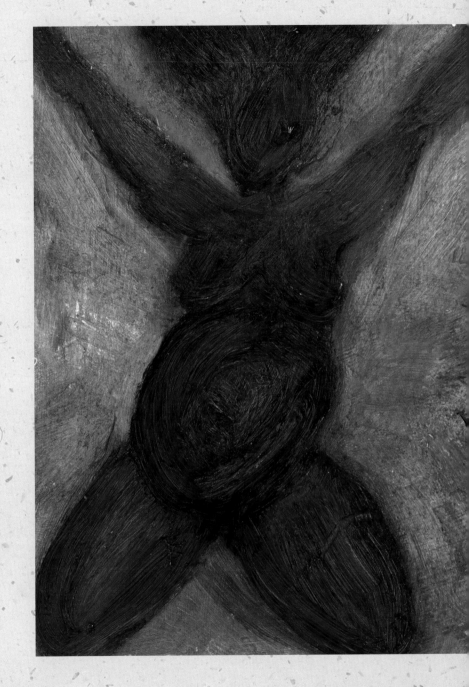

Mysticism, in its pure form, is...
union with the Absolute, and nothing else."

~ EVELYN UNDERHILL, *MYSTICISM*

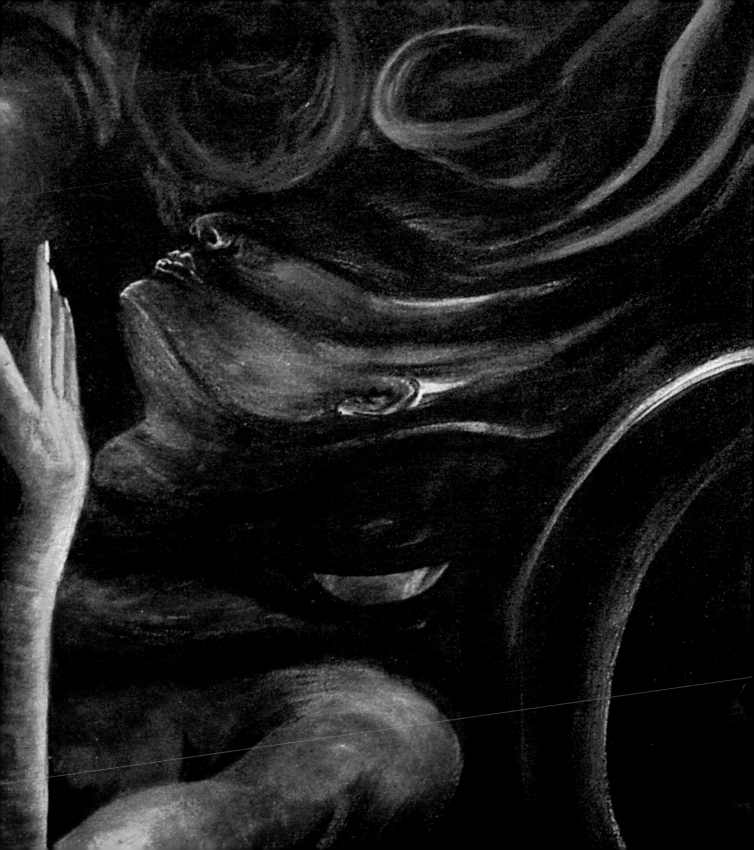

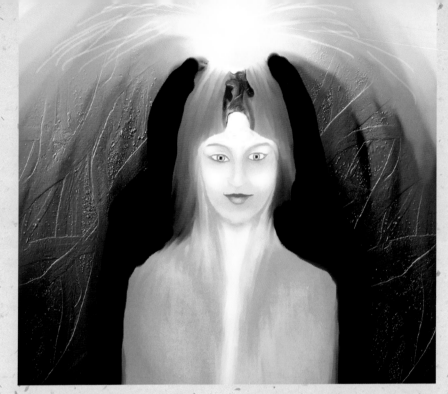

> *Mysticism means direct, immediate experience of divine reality. For Christians it's union with God. For Buddhists, it is realization of enlightenment.*
>
> – WAYNE TEASDALE,
> *THE MYSTIC HEART*

While we can buy sex and we can buy at least the trappings of religion, we can't buy, sell or trade the deep experience of spiritual-sexual union. The poetry, music, images, and stories of the love mystics make it quite clear that ecstatic experiences (eroticized and otherwise) aren't something under their control. While we human beings may be able to prevent such experiences, we certainly can't manufacture them.

It is much the same with our person-to-person sexual encounters. The particulars of a sexual encounter – the intensity and character of physical sensation, the breadth of emotional relatedness, and the spiritual depth of the experience – cannot be presupposed. Yes, we can make transcendent experiences more possible with certain preparedness, such as being present in our bodies, being psychologically integrated, and being in right relationship with our selves and each other. But the outcome – the experience itself – is beyond our control.

Spiritual-sexuality is in the realm of mystery, and such experiences are recognized by their numinous power. Spiritual sex and sexualized spirituality often include profound pleasure and something more. The more can be something like the joy of communing deeply with your lover, or a sense of being restored, or can be deeply life-affirming. In a sexualized spiritual communion, often there's a reported gift of clear-seeing, healing, and/or a new sense of purpose or direction.

BEARING FRUIT

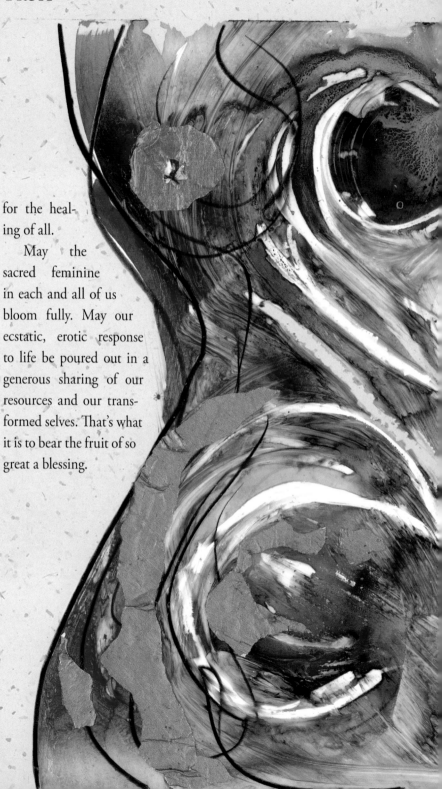

Flowering does not happen in isolation from the rest of life. The blossom time is neither the beginning nor the end, but one beautiful moment among many. Our own blossoming – our healing and unfolding as sexual-spiritual beings – matters. It matters for each of us, for each other, and for the planet.

Girls and women need role-models of healthy sexual-spiritual women.

Many children and adults need education, encouragement, and support in order to be free.

Vulnerable people of every race and gender need practical and material assistance in order to live and thrive.

Our gorgeous earth needs allies.

These are some of the places we may be called to "share the fruit" of our integrated healthy feminine spirit. An integrated healthy feminine spirit – in women and in men – seeks the healing of all – is *required* for the healing of all.

May the sacred feminine in each and all of us bloom fully. May our ecstatic, erotic response to life be poured out in a generous sharing of our resources and our transformed selves. That's what it is to bear the fruit of so great a blessing.

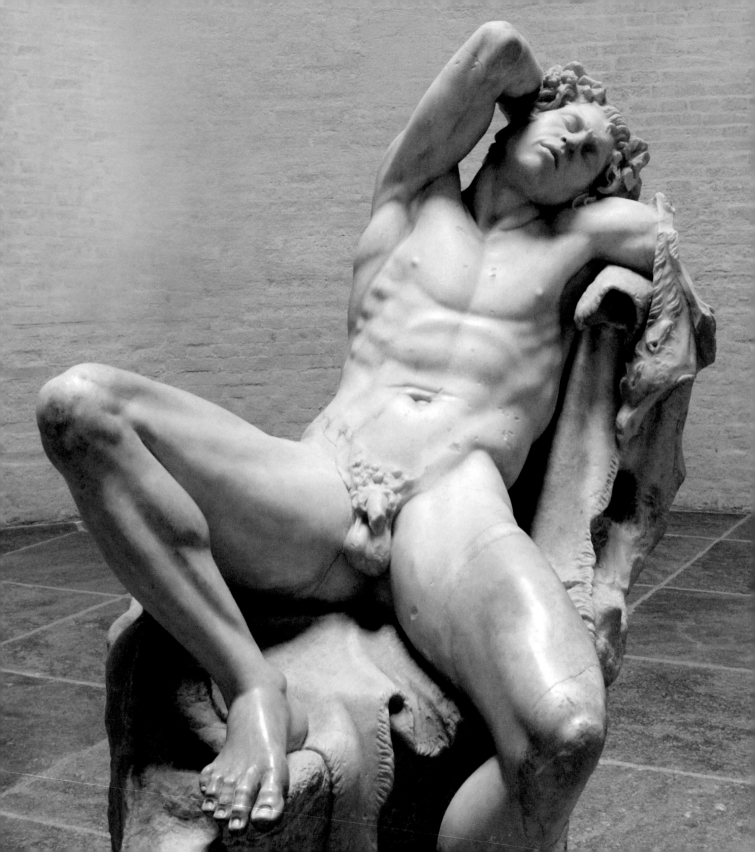

4
Male Sexuality, Masculine Spirituality

MICHAEL SCHWARTZENTRUBER

Sexual issues are always at the heart of masculine spirituality.
~ RICHARD ROHR

I'm not sure how old I was – probably eight or nine. It was a warm summer day and I was in my family's garage, although I don't remember what I was doing there. What I *do* remember is being overcome with desire. I wanted… no, I *yearned* to my core to see the naked body of the girl who lived across the street. This was not simply childhood curiosity about what she might have "down there." I had three sisters. I *knew* what she had down there. It was more than that. I felt it as a deeply sexual longing.

Which doesn't mean that I wanted sex. To be honest, I didn't know anything about sexual intercourse or about any other kind of sexual activity. But in that moment, I experienced myself as a sexual being. I experienced the power of eros, the force of attraction, and perhaps even the desire for union that drives sexuality.

At the time, I didn't comprehend any of this in a conscious way. And if the cause of my erotic yearning was a mystery to me then, I confess that it is only slightly less mysterious today. Yet I'm more aware than ever of the call of eros in my life and of myself as a sexual being. So what's up?

Myths and Misdemeanours

Popular belief asserts that men are supposed to have one-track minds when it comes to women and supposedly spend almost all their time thinking about sex. However, I suspect that many men would, like myself, have difficulty articulating what sexuality is and what it means to them, and an even harder time relating this to any notion of spirituality.

Part of the problem may be that men are just as much the victims of cultural myths and expectations – many of them contradictory – as women are. Take that notion that men have one-track minds and that sex is the only train running on it. On the one hand, everyone expects men to enjoy and want sex. On the other hand, we're not supposed to want it *too* much. But how much is too much, or not enough, and who decides? The individual man, or his partner, or the social group, or…?

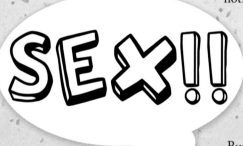

When *Globe and Mail* columnist Sarah Hampson wrote an article[1] in which she suggested that one of the primary reasons men leave their partners is because the women in-volved don't "put out" enough, and that if women want to keep their men they better be prepared to offer sex on demand… well, let's just say not everyone agreed. Especially women, many of whom wrote letters saying that, in their own relationships, *they* were the ones who wanted sex and it was their husbands who weren't interested.

The truth, of course, is that men, like women, come in all varieties when it comes to their sexual appetite. Yet the stereotype that men want sex above almost everything else persists, to the detriment of men on both ends of the libido spectrum. Those with larger sexual appetites may be judged for wanting sex *too much* and may feel that they have to walk on eggshells when it comes to their sex drive. Or they may worry that their "horniness" will be treated as self-ishness, to paraphrase one man quoted in Hampson's article. At the other end of the spectrum, men with a modest or minimal or no sex drive may worry that they will be judged "less of a man" because of it.

When it comes to male sexuality, myths and stereotypes abound. Bernie Zilbergeld, author of *The New Male Sexuality*, has com-piled the most complete – and funniest – list I've found, in a chapter he calls "It's Two Feet Long, Hard as Steel, and Will Knock Your Socks Off." The title alone points to some of the more obvious myths, but a few other examples might help fill in the picture.

- Men are liberated and comfortable with sex.
- Men aren't into stuff like feelings and communicating.
- All touching should lead to sex.
- Men are always interested in and ready for sex.
- Real men "perform."
- Sex is centred on how hard a man's penis is and what he does with it.
- A real man will make the earth move for his partner.
- Good sex is spontaneous and doesn't involve planning and talking.[2]

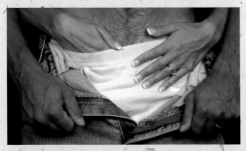

These myths seem patently absurd when you read them in a list like this. Zilbergeld actually refers to them as part of the "fantasy model of sex" depicted in everything from novels and magazines to movies and television dramas. Still, it's amazing how intertwined and entangled these ideas can become with a man's sense of identity and masculinity. If I don't live up to the sexual performances I read about or see on the screen, what kind of man does that make me? How do I separate my sense of my own sexuality – my sexual appetites, likes and dislikes, values and perspectives – from the sexual fantasy world sold as the real thing?

To complicate matters further, for the past few decades many men have been paying close attention to feminist women who have shown the devastating impact of patriarchy. As James Nelson says in his book *The Intimate Connection*, we have become aware of our sexism and of some of the "destructive aspects of the traditional male role."[3] And some of us sincerely want to change. While some men have responded to the feminist critique by becoming defensive and angry, many others have been genuinely grateful for the freedom to step away from roles and expectations that never fit them particularly well in the first place.

"Getting in touch with our feminine side" is one way men in the latter category might talk about this change. Yet this, too, can be a source of confusion and ambiguity if you have been brought up to believe that the so-called "feminine" characteristics you are now trying to embody are "inferior," as most men in the West have been taught.

In other words, figuring out what it means to be male and sexual is not an easy thing given the cultural stereotypes and myths men face, as well as the exterior and interior pressures both to resist and embrace change.

SEX, SPIRITUALITY, AND SELF-ACCEPTANCE

I have never once had a man tell me that he felt his sexuality was whole, healthy, and happy. It always seems to be a cross, a dilemma, a shame, a fear, a doubt or an impossible desire.

- RICHARD ROHR

To love oneself is the beginning of a lifelong romance.

- OSCAR WILDE

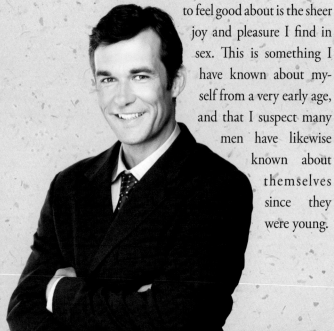

But what does any of this have to do with spirituality?

I know it's dangerous and presumptuous, not to mention impossible, to speak for all men, so let me be clear that I'm speaking only for myself when I say that *more than anything, what I want as a man is to feel good about myself and my sexuality.* I would, however, venture to say that I am not alone in this.

The ability to love and accept yourself as you are – just like the ability to forgive yourself when necessary – is bedrock when it comes to healthy spirituality. As Jesus and so many sages since have reminded us, we are called to love our neighbour *and* ourselves. More to the point, we really *can't* love our neighbour – which in the present context includes our sexual partner – if we can't first love ourselves.

One of the things I personally want to feel good about is the sheer joy and pleasure I find in sex. This is something I have known about myself from a very early age, and that I suspect many men have likewise known about themselves since they were young.

Bernie Zilbergeld describes how, on a number of occasions, he has come across a group of boys looking at a *Playboy* or *Penthouse* magazine in a bookstore. Setting aside for the moment the whole issue of erotica and pornography, how you define it and what its negative impacts might be, what strikes me is that Zilbergeld describes the actions of the boys in *positive* terms – quite a departure from the political correctness and negative judgments one often hears.

The only word that comes to mind to describe what I saw is *charming.* There's something truly wonderful about it, a lot of what I can only call good energy. I rarely sensed any disparagement of women. The same was true in my high-school days when we boys passed around novels with explicit sexual descriptions; there was desire, curiosity, and great enthusiasm, but really no ugly feelings towards girls or women. With testosterone virtually running our mind and bodies, we wanted to learn everything we could about the doing of sex, and we looked forward with great excitement and anticipation to the acts themselves.[4]

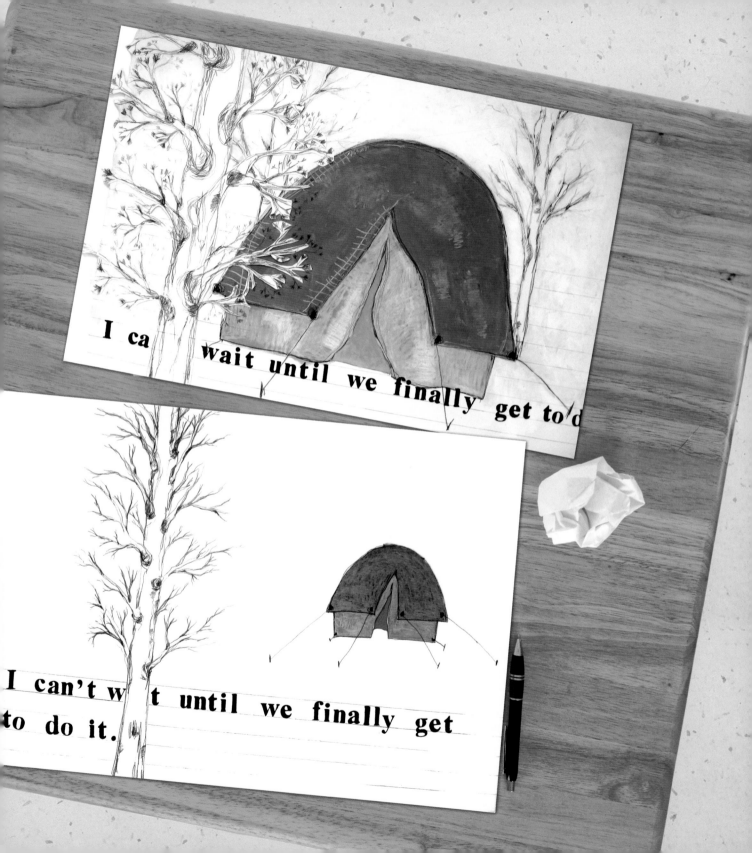

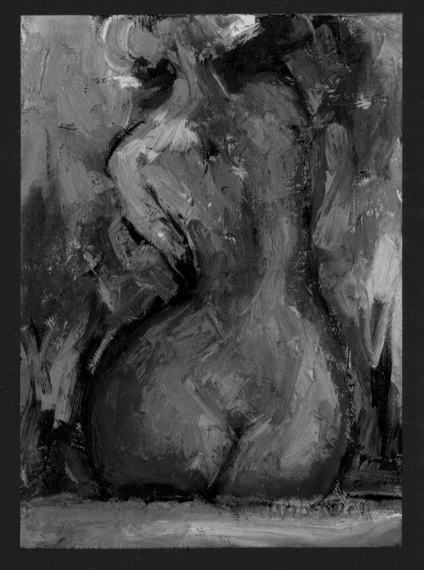

*No man is a hypocrite
in his pleasures.*

~ SAMUEL JOHNSON

To be honest, the same was true in my own experience, which mirrored Zilbergeld's in every way. The only thing I would add to Zilbergeld's description is the sense of appreciation I experienced for what I thought of then, and still think of today, as the beauty of the female form (and of the human form in general).

But I digress. The point I wanted to make is that Zilbergeld's description strikes me as both refreshing and liberating. So often, it seems, boys and men feel *guilty* about their interest in sex. There are plenty of social reasons for this. Often we experienced the judgment of parents when we were younger, or in later years the judgment of our partners, or of society.

But we are sexual beings with sexual desires, and this is something to feel good about! Something to celebrate! When we are able to do this, when we are able to affirm this central feature of our identity, we are much more likely to feel spiritually "at home" in our own skin.

HARD TRUTHS

Of course, there are other reasons many men struggle to feel spiritually at home in their bodies and with their sexuality.

It's not exactly a secret, given everything named above, that men tend to focus on their genitals as the source of their sexuality. After all, our genitals are what define us as male. James Nelson refers to this as the "genitalization" of male sexuality.

This wouldn't necessarily be a problem, except that we tend to value and focus on only one half of our genital experience – erection. And if we lose our capacity for erection? Well, let's just say it's no accident that men have spent over a billion dollars a year on Viagra since the drug first came out in 1998 – and that doesn't take into account the sales of competing products.

The ability to enjoy the physical experience of erection is incredibly important to men (and to most women, too), and rightfully so. But it goes deeper than that. Erection represents our experience of the *phallus*, which, when treated as a symbol, is often depicted as being significantly larger than life, as we saw in Chapter 2 – a pointer, perhaps, to the very large space it occupies in the male psyche.

Nelson points out that men's experience of the phallus comes in two varieties: *earthy* and *solar*.

Men encounter the earthy phallus in their experience of "sweaty, hairy, throbbing, wet, animal sexuality." We sometimes reject this part of our sexuality (and of ourselves) because it has the potential, if it becomes unbalanced, to become brutish and ugly. Yet this is life-giving energy, says Nelson, and if we deny it altogether we are left with "gentleness without strength, peacefulness without vitality, tranquility without vibrancy."

Men also experience the solar phal-

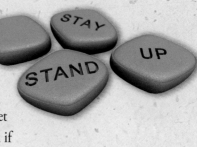

A hard man is good to find.

~ MAE WEST

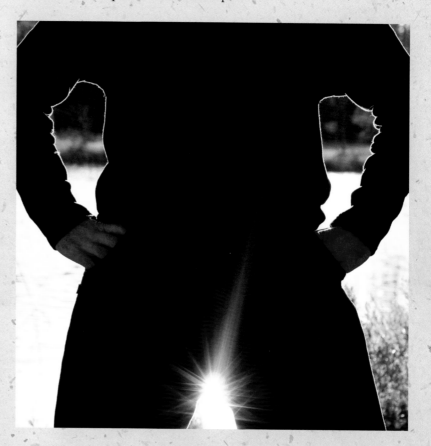

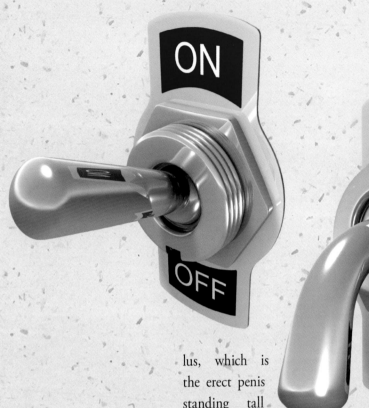

who don't "measure up"; the belief that power comes from position; the use of political influence, military power, and technical knowledge to dominate; the illusion that "bigger is better" (in paycheques, muscles, cars, buildings, corporations…); and on and on.

Once you're aware of it and begin to look, it's easy to spot both the positive and negative influences of the solar phallus, because they're everywhere.

As men, we tend to prize hardness, upness, and linearity (or straightness), and we've done a pretty thorough job of projecting these values into all areas of our lives, not just the sexual. The hard sciences and hard facts are better than the softer, less-certain people sciences and soft data. Computers and networks are "up" when they're functioning and "down" when they're not. Only "straight" men can be *real* men. For millennia, we have tended to believe that history moves in a linear fashion from past to present to future, rather than in a cyclical or spiral fashion.

And we can see this aspect of the phallus especially well in our highly patriarchal spiritual systems and religious institutions. Patriarchy is built on hierarchies and dual-

lus, which is the erect penis standing tall and proud, so to speak. Men experience the energy of the solar phallus in many aspects of their lives, not just in the bedroom. The energy behind the solar phallus is the excitement of accomplishment and strenuous achievement; it is the satisfaction of going farther physically, intellectually, and socially. The solar phallus is about transcendence, about rising above challenges, as well as above the earthy and earthly.

Like the earthy phallus, the solar phallus also has a shadow side, which shows itself as the oppression and judgment of those isms, which always imply a judgment between higher and lower (up/down), good and bad, domination and submission – and, in the religious and spiritual realm, between spirit (good) and matter (bad). Thus, a pyramid of control is erected in which

God (who is "pure spirit" and perceived in largely masculine images) must control all creation. Within creation, men (whose spirits and minds must control their own bodies and emotions) must control women (who are more bodily and emotional, deficient in reason). Adults must control children (who are less spiritual and rational in the undeveloped states). Human beings must control the soulless animals, while animals are superior to plants and plants to inorganic nature.[5]

As a result, masculine spiritualities have tended to emphasize an upward movement from the fleshly to the spiritual, from the earthy to the heavenly, with the result, says Nelson, that "holiness is tantamount to bodilessness, and saints are sexless people, mystically attuned to a life transcending earthly matter."[6]

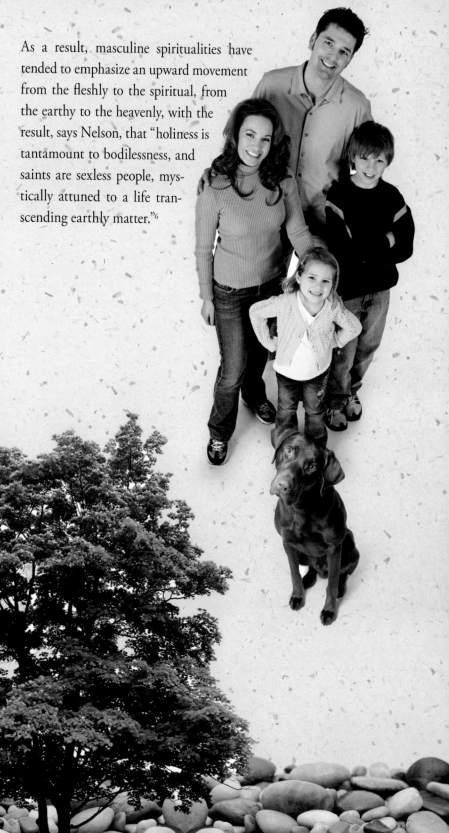

PENIS ENVY?

In other words, we've taken our keen attachment to erection and have abstracted it. We have projected onto the world a universe of phallic meanings and symbols in a process that has, ironically, largely alienated us from our actual bodily experience.

How can I say that? Well, because erection (and by extension the phallus) represents only *one half* of a man's actual genital experience. In fact, it represents much less than half. Most of the time, the penis is not erect at all, but soft. (If we were more aware, we might admit to being relieved about this. Walking around with a permanent erection would be anything but fun.) Yet we virtually ignore this fact. How can we feel at home in our bodies if we focus on only one part of our experience and ignore or treat as some kind of failure the rest?

Because that's what happens. If we can't get hard when we want to, we tend to judge ourselves harshly. We feel as if our bodies have somehow let us down.

There's a related control issue here, which we can also see in the hierarchy described on the previous page. Being "in control" – or feeling like we need to be – is such a big part of the male experience. Yet, as much as we wish we could control it, the penis seems to have a mind of its own, and often it seems like it's not paying a whole lot of attention to what's going on around it. Especially when we were younger, it would sometimes get hard when we didn't want it to. As we age, we're more likely to experience the opposite problem – a penis that remains soft when we want it to get hard.

It's difficult for a man to feel at home in his body when it doesn't do what he wants it to, when he can't control it.

The male knows the ups and downs of desire partly through his penis, and the ordinary state of being limp is as important as arousal. To be always tumescent is an undesirable condition, whether in the actual penis or in the emotions of desire and excitement.

\- Thomas Moore

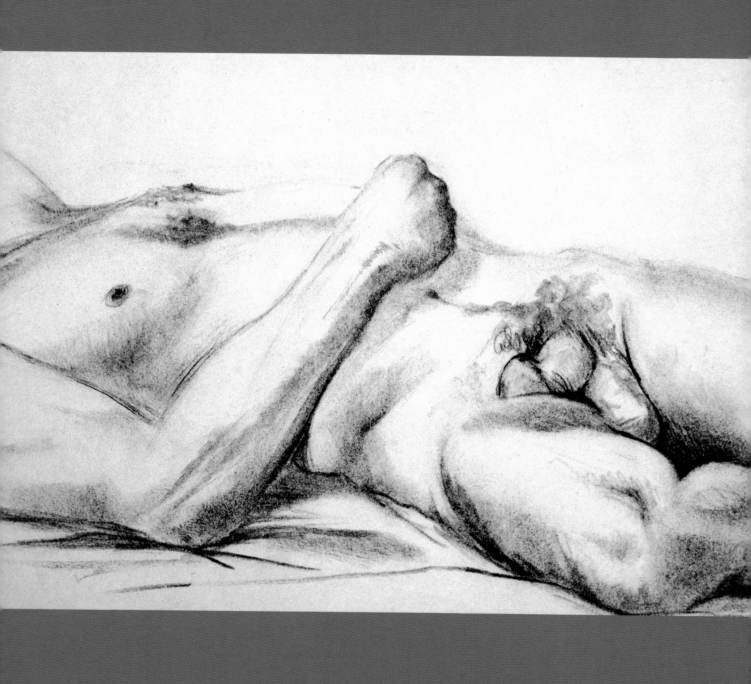

The Via Positiva and the Via Negativa

Our desire to control that which seems beyond control and our tendency to focus on only one part of our sexual experience and ignore the rest – none of this is a recipe for success if we hope to reclaim our sexuality, and find a way back into our bodies to recover the spiritual home we have there.

What men need is a more balanced perspective on their sexual experience, sexuality, and spirituality. While we need to admit the physical pleasure of erection and the positive psychic and spiritual energy of the phallus, we need also to acknowledge the reality of the soft penis, and become aware of the unique psychic and spiritual gifts it represents.

Nelson speaks about this balance in terms of the *Via Positiva* and the *Via Negativa* – the two traditional paths to God in Western spirituality.

The former is a way of affirmation, of thanksgiving, of ecstasy. It is the way of light, the way of being filled by the sacred fullness and rising to the divine height. The Via Negativa is a way of emptying and being emptied. It is the way of darkness. It is sinking into nothingness and into the sacred depths. In spirituality, each way needs the other for balance and completion. The overdevelopment of one to the detriment of the other brings distortion. I believe the male experience of the Via Positiva has profound associations with the phallus, while the Via Negativa correspondingly is connected to the [soft] penis. And in most men it is the latter which remains underrecognized, underclaimed, underaffirmed.[7]

Despite the fact that we spend more hours living with the penis than we do with the phallus, there are plenty of reasons why the penis – and the associated spiritual and psychic benefits we might gain by acknowledging it – goes "underrecognized, underclaimed, underaffirmed." Compared to an erection and the sense of urgency that goes with it, the penis is relatively undemanding and easy to ignore. It is quiet. Restful. Unobtrusive. We also tend to associate erections with youth and vitality – desirable qualities in a youth-obsessed culture – whereas we associate the soft penis with aging and impotence.

Yet the benefits of a more balanced approach to our sexuality and spirituality are real and within our grasp, if we open ourselves to them. On a purely physical level, when our penis doesn't perform as we wish it would, maybe we could relax a bit and acknowledge that this, too, is part of what it means to be male and sexual. In those times, maybe we could remember that there are many paths to intimacy and sexual pleasure, and that erection is only one of them.

And while the vital spiritual energy of the phallus is something we never want to have to give up or lose, we might find spiritual and sexual healing by recognizing the virtues of the penis and the Via Negativa. For this is the place where we can rest in the quiet stillness of the soul, in the dark interior places. Just as the penis at rest empties itself of blood, we can empty ourselves of our concerns and our need to achieve, and rest instead "in the depth of meanings we do not create."[8] Just as we must allow the penis to rest in order to experience erection, we must allow ourselves periods of spiritual quietude and regeneration so that we can live creatively and productively in the world.

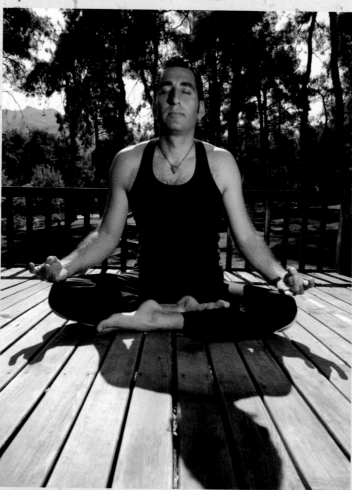

*Nothing
in all creation
is so like God
as stillness.
We are to sink
eternally
from letting go
into letting go
into God.*

~ MEISTER ECKHART

103

LOST AND FOUND

If we experience a feeling of being a bit "lost" in this unfamiliar place, well, that too may be a central feature of masculine spirituality, and by extension male sexuality.

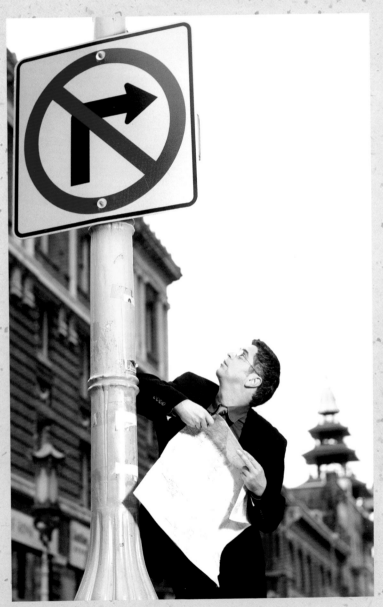

I first encountered this idea at a large gathering of church people several years ago, where David Giuliano, then Moderator of the United Church of Canada, was speaking about masculine spirituality.

For me, David's statement that men *need* the experience of being lost was one of those "Aha!" moments. Forget all those jokes about men being unwilling to ask for directions. Call it the desert or wilderness experience or whatever you will. In a very real and deeply spiritual way, men need the experience of being lost, if only so they can discover their ability to *find* their own way, or alternatively, have the experience of being *found*.

I now believe this is so true of masculine spirituality that if we don't intentionally and consciously create opportunities for this kind of experience through ritual or other means, then we will create them in a variety of unconscious ways – sometimes life-enhancing and sometimes life-destructive. Men's experience of sex and sexuality, in particular, provides ample opportunities for both.

Obviously, men have sex for a variety of reasons: to enjoy intimacy and share love, to experience physical pleasure and the release of orgasm, to relieve stress and escape boredom, to feel the excitement and vitality of arousal. All of these have their place in a balanced and healthy sex life.

Yet like all good things, sex can lead to trouble if it gets out of hand. Certainly it is possible and not uncommon for men to lose themselves in negative and destructive ways to sex, through sex addiction or addiction to pornography. We can become truly lost to our authentic selves and to those we love. And while we may learn some valuable spiritual and life lessons during these "wilderness" times, or while on the road to recovery, the damage we do to our relationships and ourselves is not small or inconsequential.

But sex can also be a vehicle through which men "lose" themselves in much more positive and generative ways. In the sacred intimacy of sex, we can cast off our inhibitions and negative self-judgments; we can let go of our ego needs and boundaries. We can die to our "small self" and become alive to our "larger self," the self that is connected to all things. As we go deep into our physical experience, we may paradoxically experience transcendence as we merge, body and spirit, with our beloved, and perhaps with all that is.

This is a deep form of losing indeed. Yet in this "lostness" we may discover our true nature as incarnate spirit. We may have the experience both of being found by the "other," and of finding our true selves.

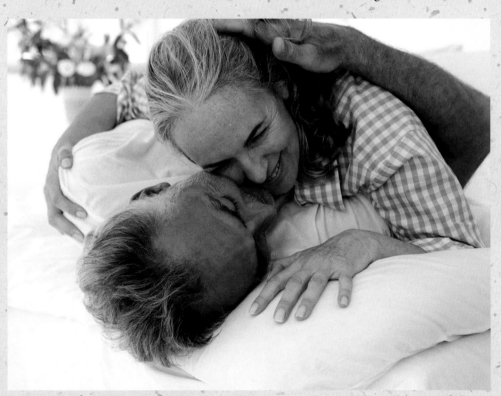

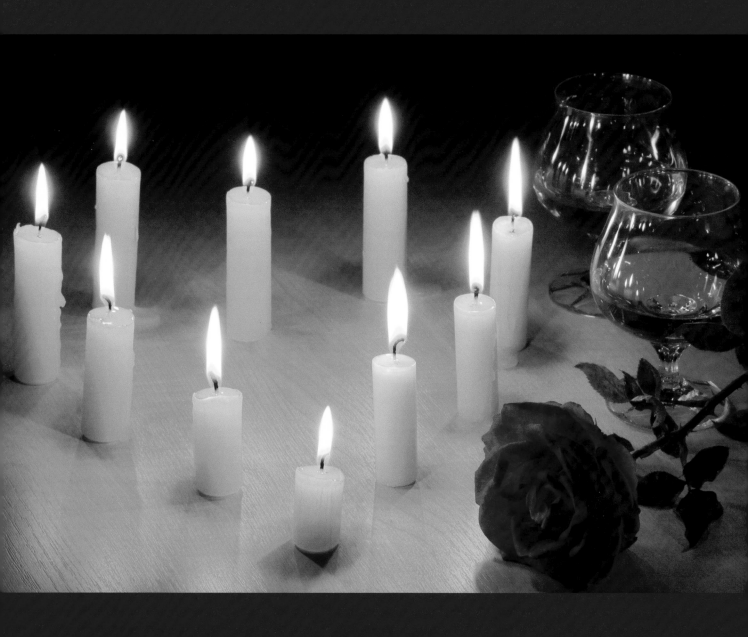

5
Sense and Sensuality

MARY MILLERD

We live in a sense luscious world, thrilling,
pampering and learning through our senses.
— DIANE ACKERMANN

The word *sensuality* elicits sighs and murmurs from me as I imagine receiving a massage, or eating chocolates, or smelling a rose, or seeing a beautiful landscape, or hearing a piece of music that touches my heart and melts my resistance. But not everyone imagines what I do when hearing the word sensuality.

I looked sensuality up in several dictionaries. Over and over again, sensuality is viewed in a dim light. It is usually described as gratification of, preoccupation with, or indulgence in appetites. It is judged as deficient in moral, spiritual or intellectual interests. Synonyms for sensuality are voluptuous, worldly, and irreligious. I was relieved

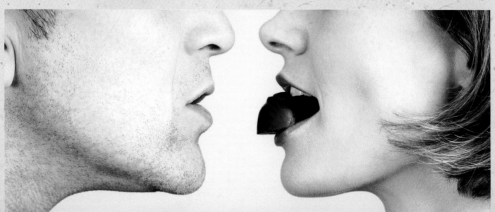

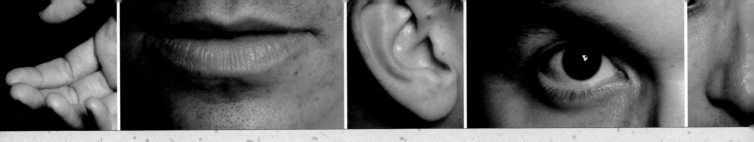

when I read in the *Concise Oxford English Dictionary* that a more traditional usage of the word sensual is "relating to the senses rather than the intellect" – although it did acknowledge in a highlighted note that the word is usually used to refer to gratifying the senses, especially in a sexual way.

No wonder our bodies get such a bad rap, particularly in some religious communities. Our senses are seen by many as having little to do with our spiritual lives. With the above definition in mind, a person might even say senses are a distraction from the spiritual life, and are therefore bad.

Fortunately, although this view of sensuality may still be the predominant one in our culture, it is not the only view.

Take a moment and say or think the word: *sensuality*. What is your response to the word? Does it make you feel uncomfortable? Does it excite you? Do you wish your response was different? Notice the thoughts you have. Notice your desire to experience the word. Drop deeper into your body and feel the word. Then find the words to describe what you are feeling. What does sensuality feel like to you?

When I focus on sensuality, my body relaxes. I breathe more deeply. I feel luscious and warm. I experience a communion of the parts of myself: body, spirit, emotions.

My thoughts are quite different. My thoughts reveal that I am afraid of what my mother and father will think of me. And what my children will think of me when they find out I'm a sexual being. This is all okay. This is what is, and from this place of awareness I can choose something new – in this case, more room for sensuousness.

Sensuality is about resonance. Whenever we see, hear, taste, smell, and touch in an attentive way, we "feel" in our body what some would call a "felt sense." Eugene Gendlin describes it as "an internal aura that encompasses everything you feel."[1] It is a deep knowing of what the experience is for us. We feel first, and then we find words to describe what we are feeling. Like when we are in love, a simple glance into our beloved's eyes can elicit waves of sensations in our body that leave us speechless. We long to communicate what we are feeling.

Our senses are an integral part of how we communicate. Our senses connect us

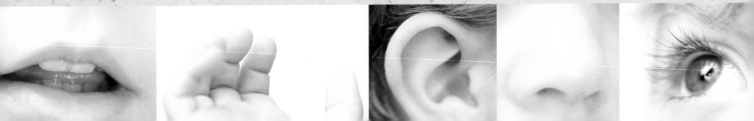

with the outer world, gathering information for us to experience. Our senses keep us connected to our own body, our own experience, and our response to our experience. Through our senses we can be aware of our lover's body and their senses, what they like and don't like. As we stay in the moment with each other, mingling through our senses, where giving pleasure is receiving pleasure, we can communicate our love and longing for each other – an embodied experience of "the spirit in me greets the spirit in you."

Our senses are not bad. They are essential to a rich and full life. It is through our senses that we come to know our spiritual presence, to know ourselves as incarnate beings. We can feel spirit flowing within us. Thomas Keating calls spirit the "river of consciousness."[2] The "great river" is our underlying fundamental entity, a part of God, our essential and emergent self.

Beatrice of Nazareth, a 13th-century ecstatic mystic, writes about the "manner of love" in which "the soul experiences sweetness, freedom and delight when 'it feels all its senses sanctified in love.'"[3] Hadewijch, a 14th-century Beguine nun, "describes how the loved one and the Divine Lover dwell in each other in such a way 'that neither of the two distinguishes himself from the other... while one sweet divine nature flows through them both, and they are both one

thing through each other, but at the same time both remain – yes, and remain so forever.'"[4] Beatrice and Hadewijch are making love with God. Their sexual experience is celibate, yet does not lack sensuality. It is luscious. Imagine sharing this love, this sex, with another.

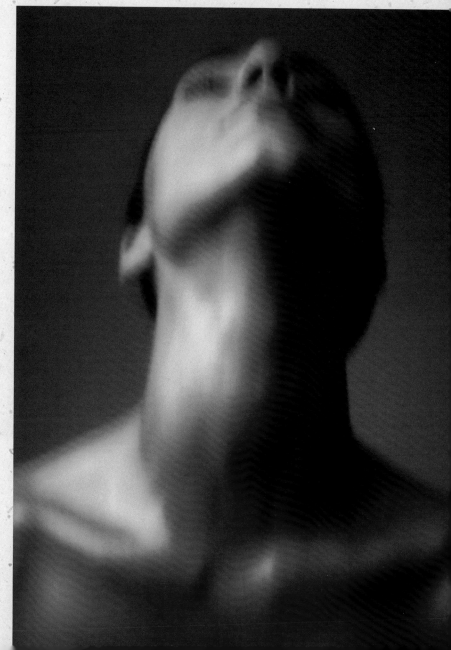

Our Inner Lover

To be sensual or sensuous is to be in the presence of your own soul.

~ John O'Donohue

Great lovemaking has a lot to do with how we feel about ourselves. How we feel about ourselves affects our ability to experience our wholeness in the body, our intimate and sacred space. Eros is about wholeness. It is a unifying energy within us, in relationships and in societies. Eros is experienced by many as a rush of energy in the body that lifts us up out of sluggishness, causing the sensitivity of the body to increase, creating a luscious, sensuous feeling of pleasure and well-being. Our sensuality is our body's felt sense of eros, our *inner lover*.

Are you aware of a lover inside of you, whispering lovingly in your ear how much you are adored no matter what you are doing or what is going on? Your inner lover can help you remember what needs to be done, hold you accountable, keep life light,

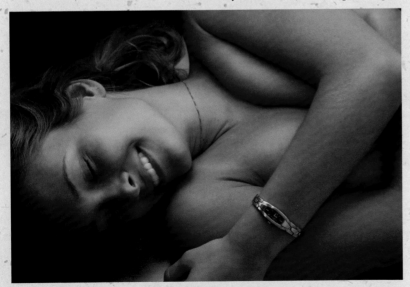

and come up with new ideas so you don't get stuck or bored.

Perhaps you are more aware of the critic inside of you, who punishes you when you forget or make a mistake, who makes work hard rather than fun, scrunching your creativity.

Both our inner lover and critic have their own energy that resonates in our body and affects our well-being. My inner lover softens me and opens me to experience my life. I resist my inner critic, becoming defensive, anxious, and overly careful. Whichever is stronger at the moment resonates within me. People who are empathetic can often pick up the resonance of others. Sometimes they can feel it in their own bodies and sometimes they simply see the tension or relaxation in another's body. Listening to our inner lover helps us to stay in tune with our own experience and helps us set the tone in our relationships with others.

How we talk to ourselves, how we treat ourselves in our struggles and joys affects our sensuality. What supports us to be sensual, sense-filled people? Safety. Before we open ourselves to our sensuousness, we need to feel safe.

Safety will vary from person to person. The biggest factor is judgment, and we are usually our own worst critics. We fear judgment and brace ourselves against it. Am I doing it right? Do I look stupid? Am I attractive? Our judgments shut down our sensuality, our ability to sense ourselves from the inside. Without the sensuousness flowing within us, we feel fragmented and look to others for approval. Our sense of our own inner beauty and our light and truth is dimmed and people cannot see us.

Our Western culture's focus on beauty as an outward quality fails to support us in knowing and embracing our inner beauty, which is a spiritual quality. There is nothing more attractive than a person who loves and cares for themselves. There is nothing more beautiful than someone showing their beauty, their vulnerability, their soul. They shine, they glow, they are engaging and interesting, and they are engaged and interested in us.

When we trust our inner lover to translate our own and others' judgments to information that helps us, we feel safe. With safety we can relax, sit back within ourselves, and feel the sensations – our sensuality.

Our sensations happen in the moment. If we get lost in our thoughts, we can let our inner lover gently bring us back to the present moment simply by paying attention to our sensations. When we are present to our own sensuality, we bring eros in our midst, a wonderful start to lovemaking.

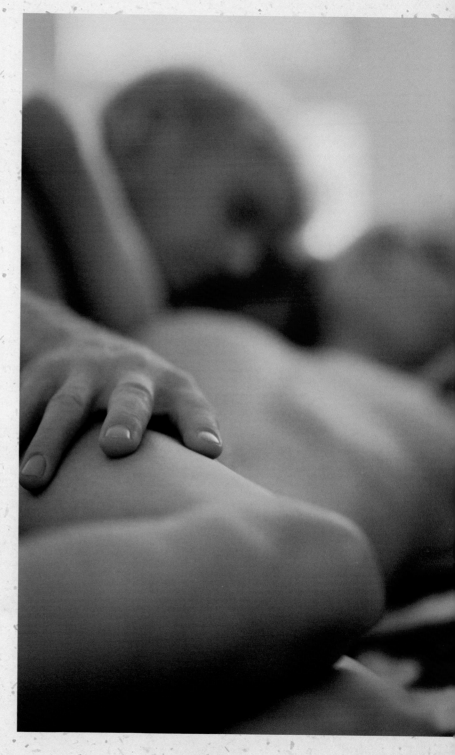

Falling in Love

Our first full experience of our sensuality happens to many of us when we fall in love and eros takes hold of us. We are overwhelmed by what we are feeling. We are full of passion and anguish. We feel the tension of opposites, never wanting it to end and longing to be fulfilled. Often, we can't eat, sleep, or do anything without thoughts of our lover and what we'd like to do with them. Whatever we have not "done" we fantasize about, imagining every detail of a possible encounter. Our fantasies are enough for the floodgates of our sensuality to burst open. Sometimes we don't know which way is up. We feel confused, and we simply long to take our beloved to bed and have our way.

How we navigate our experience of falling in love and the compelling force of eros will be an individual response. We may lose

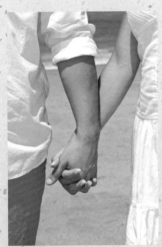

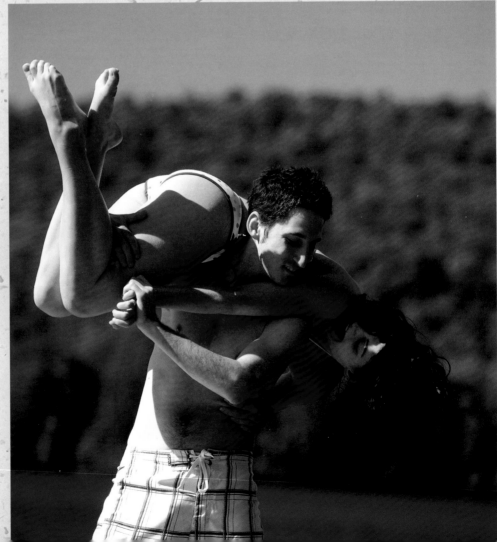

touch with our inner lover and focus on the object of our attraction. Many of us will feel the intensity of our arousal so much that we will want to rush into having sex to break the sensual tension that our body is experiencing. We may believe our powerful erotic response is true love. Sometimes it is, and sometimes it isn't. The compelling nature of eros can get us into trouble if we lose our ability to choose our response from a place of integrity within ourselves.

Others will savour the erotic tension, wanting to explore the connection emotionally and intellectually before they explore it sexually. Staying connected with their own inner lover, they are able to contain the intensity of the arousal of their sensuality. Contain does not mean constrain or repress. It means we have the capacity to feel intensely and not be controlled by what we are feeling. We are able to maintain a sense of ourselves and not get lost in our sensations. Our body does not take over, but we are present in our fullness of body, emotion, mind, and spirit. When we are ready to make love, we are aware of our inner lover. We are aware of the intensity of our arousal, and we are aware of this in our lover. Spiritual presence in our lovemaking supports us to surrender to it, a transformative experience.

Many discover in an exploration of sexuality an expanded realm of the senses which has the power to lead them from the occasionally ridiculous to the often sublime. They recognize that the wholehearted investigation of their sexuality is essential if their bond is to become a mystical union.

– Stephen and Ondrea Levine

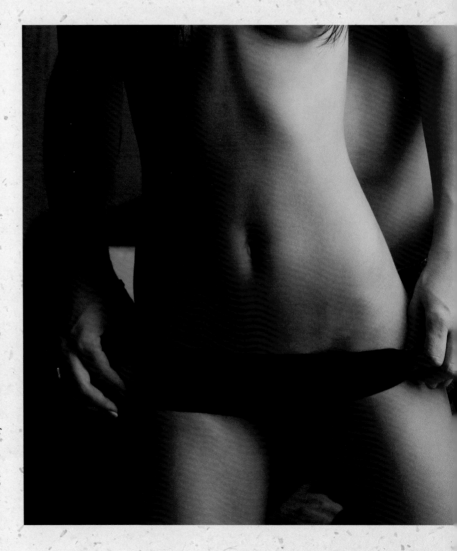

Your senses link you intimately with the divine within you and around you.
- JOHN O'DONOHUE

Sexuality is the way we are intimate with our own feeling states; the way we are moved by the diamonds of rain on a spider web; our paintings and letters; our laughter and stews; our persuasions and politics. Sexuality is our moment-by-moment, changing relish for who we are. Sexuality is our willingness to let ourselves really show in the world.

-JALAJA BONHEIM

All of life is interconnected. Our sensuality and our sexuality are vital parts of our connection with our humanity and with humanity. Many of us struggle to find a balance between our individuality (a feeling of being alone) and our connectivity (a feeling of oneness or "we-ness"[5]) in our relationships. Sex is one expression of our desire for loving connection.

I grew up in the sixties in the era of "free love." That time flowed with erotic energy and a lot of sexual experimentation. The need to know someone well before having sex wasn't always necessary. When I talk to my children, who are in their twenties and thirties, they tell me that there is a lot of ease around sex these days also.

One of my younger friends is not partnered, but still longs to share her sensuality, her sense of self, and her eroticism with another. She has a few friends she can call who help meet her sexual needs. These relationships are what's known as "friends with benefits." I am aware of the dignity my friend brings to these encounters. I'm also aware of her sadness, for she longs for a committed relationship. Until she meets someone, she will fuel her spiritual and erotic connection with her body by having sex with her friends.

Others I know have chosen celibacy, at least temporarily. Celibacy is not about a lack of sexuality or sensuality. Celibacy is the choice not to act on one's sexual, sensuous desires by having sex with another. Some people choose celibacy for religious reasons, to deepen their relationship with the Beloved, with God. Some people choose celibacy because one of their principles is not to have sex outside of a committed relationship. To cross their principles compromises their sense of dignity and integrity.

Whether we are celibate, have "friends with benefits," or are in a committed relationship, being connected with our inner lover helps us feel good about ourselves. We feel it as a resonance in our body. A part of feeling good is feeling our sensuality, and so a part of our self-care is being mindful of our sensual self. Creating opportunities for ourselves to nurture our relationship with our inner lover helps us to be good lovers with others. Exploring our own body through all of our senses helps us to feel safe inside of ourselves.

When we learn the language of our own body and trust what it tells us, we don't have to fake it. We don't have to make ourselves do what we don't want to do. We also don't have to stop ourselves from doing what feels right for us. We can be spiritually present in and with our bodies and share the wonder of ourselves with another.

Preparing for Our Lover

A romantic evening with our lover is a journey. We make physical and emotional space to welcome, invite, rest, nourish, refresh, and delight in each other through our senses. When you are planning a romantic evening with your lover, consider what you might do to arouse an awareness of your senses.

Since what we see is often our first conscious contact with an experience (and also impacts how we feel on the inside), pay attention to what your lover will see in your home. Walk around your home from your own point of view as well as your lover's and see if it supports the feeling you want for your romantic evening. Do this even if your lover lives with you and is very familiar with the space. Make it new by freshening it up.

Glance around and notice what your lover will see upon arrival. An uncluttered entranceway gives a feeling of spaciousness. Spaciousness helps us to relax and feel safe. You may have a painting or a piece of art that is welcoming or restful, that puts you and others at ease in your home. Plants also help to do this. Or a few bouquets of flowers strategically located around your home can warm the welcome.

Take this same eye to the rest of the spaces you and your lover will share. Move things around until you are satisfied with how the rooms make you feel. Flowers, candles, and dimmed light can evoke a soft, intimate atmosphere that invites you both into an emotional, erotic connection. If you have a bathtub for two or a hot tub, consider taking a beverage with you and having a lovely, relaxing soak together. A scented soak relaxes and soothes, enhancing sensuality.

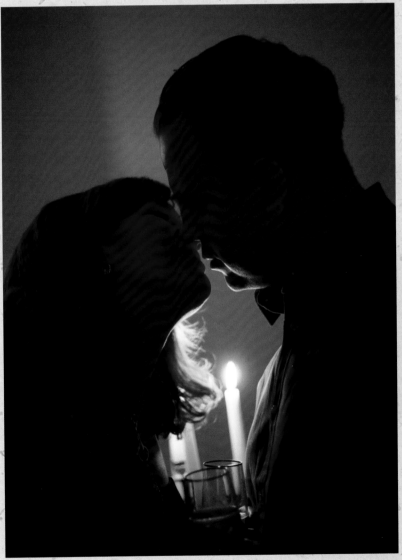

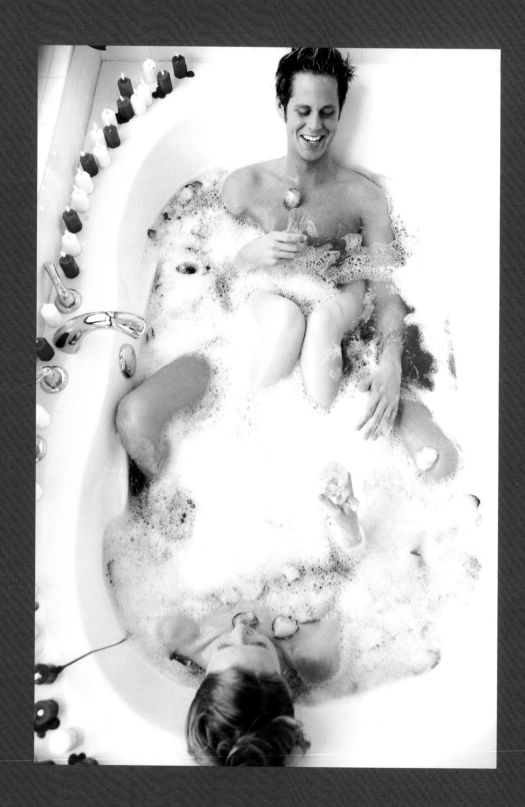

Attend particularly to the room in which you plan to make love. At the same time, remain open to being surprised – perhaps the living room or the kitchen would be delicious places to savour each other's bodies. On the other hand, you may want to sequester yourselves in the bedroom, where you can feel the intimacy of a smaller space. Be mindful of the sheets you choose, the pillows that are available, and the lighting you will use. Again, check the room through your own sensual experience. Does the room support the feeling, the resonance with your lover, that you want? If the rooms are inviting to you, chances are your lover will feel it too.

Music affects our emotions. Our internal state of being will often resonate at the emotional tone of the music we are listening to. Consider the music you will play when your lover arrives, while you are preparing a meal, eating, and sipping wine together. Think about the kind of music that moves an emotional connection to a sexual connection. What music brings closure to a beautiful evening?

A meal is often part of a romantic evening. Having something that smells delicious cooking when your lover arrives can be very inviting and relaxing. Have a glass of your lover's favourite beverage ready and waiting. Choose foods that energize you,

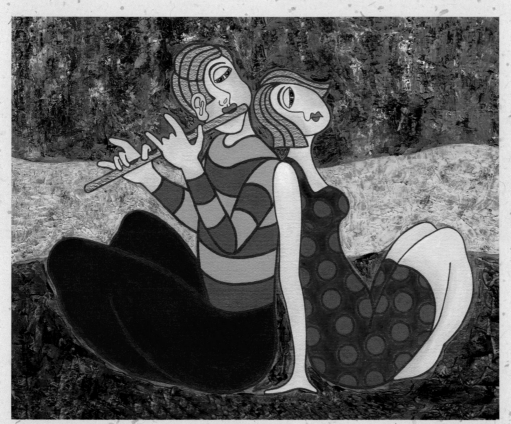

The ear is the road to the heart.

~ VOLTAIRE

make you feel fresh inside and out, foods that smell, look, and taste delicious.

And then there's touch. Ah... lovely touch. It arouses so many feelings in us, both emotional and physical. A simple gesture, touching a shoulder or an arm, can send shivers of delight through our whole body. How we touch each other, whether having sex or not, is a part of lovemaking. As innocent as it may seem, it can be electric. Through touch we can create a vibrational or resonant connection that moves us into sync with each other. We become aware of each other's state of being, each other's emotions, and we feel known. When our lovemaking moves in this way, it simply unfolds; no planning is necessary. It seems we just know what to do.

Creating an environment that helps us and our lover to feel our bodies through our senses is one of the ways we prepare ourselves for our lover. A relaxed and open environment helps us to be relaxed and open. Nurturing our senses through sight, sound, smell, taste, and touch softens and enlivens us at the same time. A delicious environment where sensuality flourishes invites an erotic connection, and sometimes a sexual one as well.

It was not my lips you kissed, but my soul.
- JUDY GARLAND

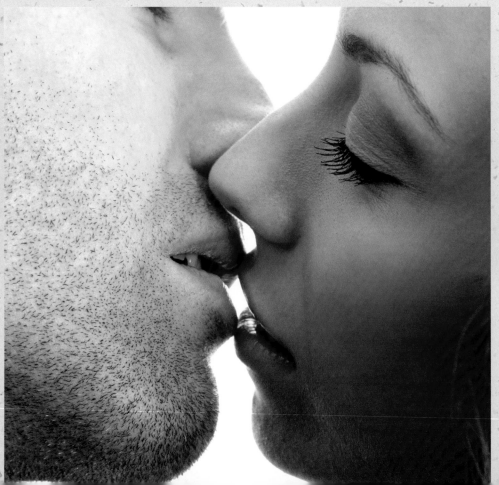

Preparing for Spiritual Sex

Our relationship with ourselves is a basic ingredient for our sexual encounters. It sets the tone, influencing our inner and outer environments. When we are relaxed, we settle our mind and open our heart, and we connect within ourselves. We are able to feel our sensuality. When we feel sensuous in the presence of others, it creates intimacy.

"Hugging till relaxed,"[6] coined by David Schnarch, author of *Passionate Marriage,* is a practice that helps us to feel our sensuality with our lover. Hugging till relaxed allows us to connect with each other without the distraction of sex, and prepares us for a connection during sex which opens us to knowing each other deeply. There are many techniques that help us to relax, but I have found hugging till relaxed most effective, because it involves touching another person spiritually and physically. It is one way we integrate spirituality and sexuality.

Schnarch does not give specific instructions on how to hug till relaxed. He does encourage us to explore what helps us to relax and to feel our sensuality. The intent is to hug with our lover until we can simply be present to "what is," free of tension and free of expectation.

I have found that hugging till relaxed has similar elements to mindful meditation. Focusing on my own sensations, I feel grounded and centred. I feel spiritually present and available. With my inner lover I mindfully scan my body, noticing where my muscles are tense and where they are slack. I breathe into the tense muscles, inviting them to let go and relax. I breathe into the slack muscles to energize them. As I relax, I often feel a release and fullness in my body, followed by a deep breath. This seems to be a natural place for the hug to end.

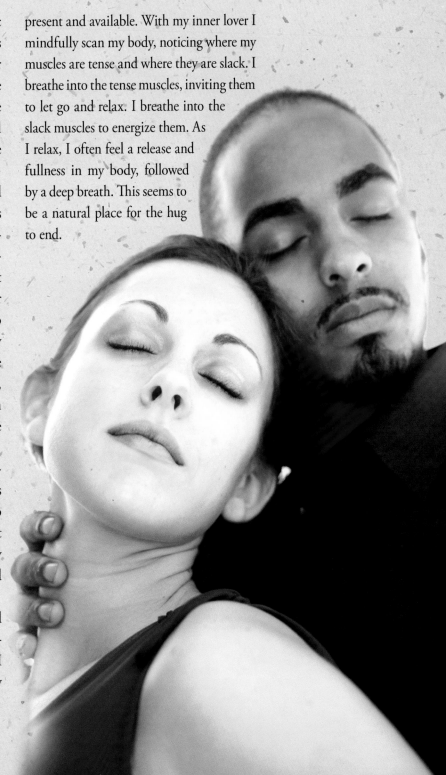

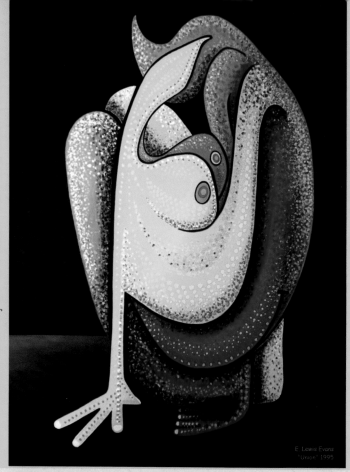

E. Lewis Evans
'Union' 1995

Allowing ourselves to consider relaxing reveals to us our inner state of being. Do we want to know how we are feeling? Can we stay with our own emotional and sensate experience without distracting ourselves? Do we feel safe or defensive? Do we relax or tense up? Does our mind wander, waiting for the hug to end? Are we enduring it? How relaxed can we let ourselves be?

When we relax, we can feel ourselves, our own inner experience to an outer event. We can feel the sensate information our body picks up. We can feel our emotions and sensations, which connect us deeply and erotically with ourselves.

From a solid stance of being tuned in to ourselves, we can then tune in to – resonate with – our partner, connecting deeply, a connection we cannot fake. To explore and touch each other's bodies without physically exploring and touching creates an erotic, emotional connection. No sacrifices need be made to fulfill one's own desires or to relieve the pressure of a lover's expectations. Hugging while relaxed opens us to a different experience of sacrifice. Instead

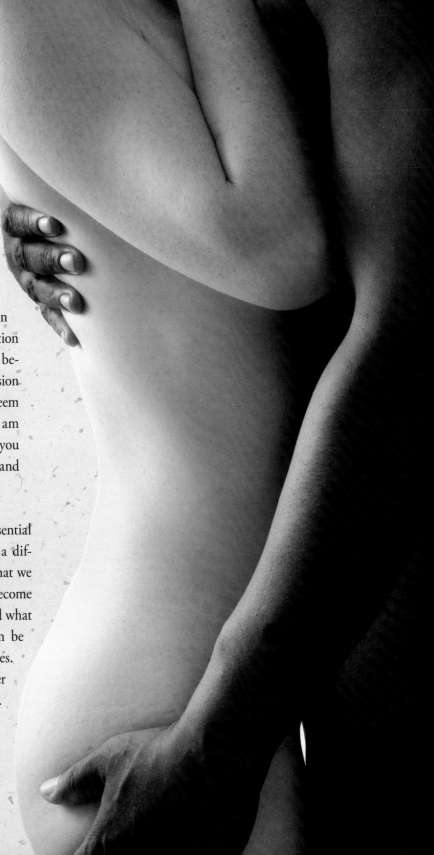

of feeling like we are losing something, our experience is of receiving. We hug to feel ourselves in the presence of another. John Haule says it beautifully.

> The structure of erotic interaction...makes it fairly clear that the call of Eros discernible in our we-ness can be heard and responded to only when the two of us can maintain both our own separate integrity and our participation in the unity that comes to presence between us. The urge to abort the tension between the I and the we may seem more than we can bear. But when I am able to bear this tension, I enable you to come to presence in your full and unique otherness.[7]

Hugging till relaxed reveals our essential and emergent self, and opens us to a different level of communication, one that we might call communion. We may become aware of both what we are feeling and what our partner is feeling. So much can be said with a gesture or a look in our eyes. We feel the meaning of what another is communicating to us in our body. Learning the language of our body takes time.

Dismantling Roadblocks

Relaxing is not as easy as one would think or hope. David Schnarch writes about how anxiety and muscle tension block our experience of sensuality. Decreased sensuality lowers desire, decreases self-knowledge, and prevents us from deeply connecting with each other. All of us tend to have a baseline of tension. It is a feeling of being ready to respond. We are relaxed while hugging when our tension is below our baseline. Hugging till relaxed calms us and deepens our connection with ourselves and others.

Many people are afraid to relax because they fear losing their sense of self. They don't feel they can trust their lover. Yet if we can't feel ourselves, if we do not know and trust our own sensuality, we cannot trust another. We need to begin within ourselves, by learning the language of our own body.

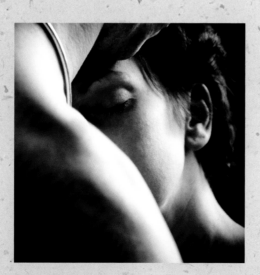

Others are afraid to relax because relaxation helps us to feel our sensations and emotions. Some people find the experience uncomfortable. They prefer to keep their emotions at a distance, which keeps their sensuality at a distance as well.

Hugging till relaxed creates a level of relaxation that helps us to purify our senses. In the process, memories may surface and images may come to mind – old wounds or anxieties. As we stay with our sensations, we can let our thoughts, memories, and images float by, releasing them so we can stay emotionally present with ourselves and our lover. As we let go and settle into ourselves in the presence of another, we can hear the quiet. We may find our breathing synchronizes with our lover's. In this way, hugging till relaxed helps us heal, resolving the past in the present.

It is important to have our inner lover with us while hugging till relaxed. If any of our self-trashing surfaces, our inner lover can put it in its place. Staying with our sensations helps us to stay out of judgment and stay in present time, in the moment. Simply be mindful of what you feel. If you are not feeling your sensations or feeling some kind of connection (eros) with the person you are hugging, chances are you are holding yourself back. Resting in our inner lover opens us to tune back in to ourselves.

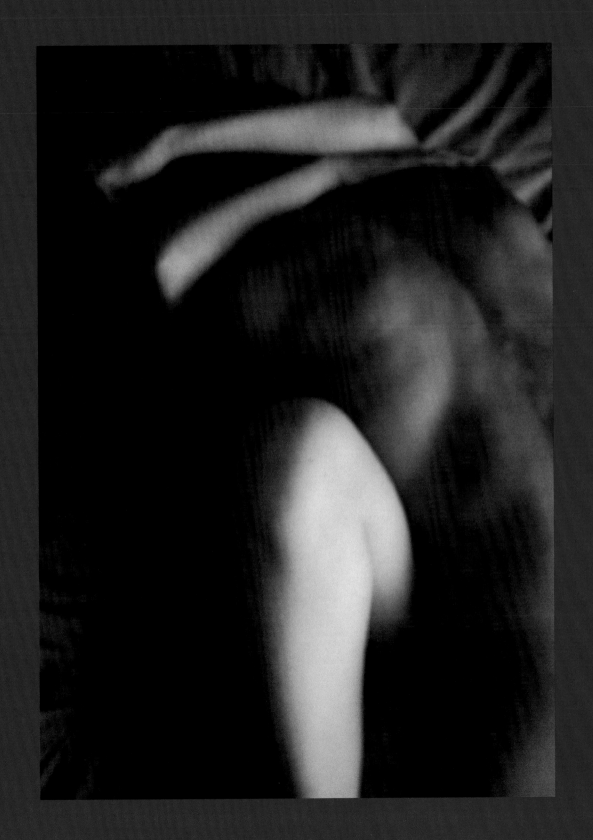

GOING WITH THE FLOW

The instinct, rhythm and radiance of the human body come alive vividly when we make love. We slip down into a more ancient penumbral rhythm where the wisdom of the body claims its own grace, ease and joy.

— JOHN O'DONOHUE

As we learn to relax while hugging, we may want to use it in our lovemaking as well. The intention of hugging till relaxed is to have a full sense of ourselves, to feel fully and deeply. It moves our lovemaking from being about technique and position to "going with the flow." With technique and position, we are focused on the outside. We can go through the moves but not necessarily be connected with what we are doing, which means there is a lack of eros and sensation. Bringing our sense of self into each move we make calms us and deepens

our connection to where eroticism becomes electric.

Going with the flow, we are focused on the inside. This does not mean we tune out our partner to focus only on our own sensations. Going with the flow is an experience where giving is receiving and receiving is giving. Like Hadewijch's mystical love experience with God, "neither of the two distinguishes himself from the other... while one sweet divine nature flows through them both, and they are both one thing through each other, but at the same time both remain."

Sándor Ferenczi, a follower of Freud, said that "sex is a return to the oceanic sensation of the infant in the womb." Like a baby in the womb, we create a bubble of energy around us that alters our consciousness and focuses us on our lover only. Through our senses, we mingle with and in each other spiritually and physically. We drink each other in with our eyes, in awe of what we behold in the other, smelling, tasting and touching each other, revealing our vulnerable and tender self – deep communion. It is a place of trust and deep knowing. So much is said with no words at all, except perhaps a sigh or a moan. We touch to affirm the realness of the other, that they are present, heart and soul. Sex makes our love for each other manifest. We make love spiritually and physically – there is no separation.

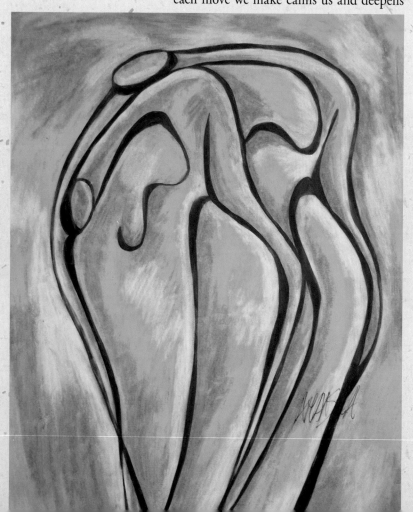

Namaste

The experience of spiritual sex varies from person to person; it varies within a relationship. Our sensuality is fundamental to it. Our senses are the bridge between our inner and outer worlds. Our senses let us know about ourselves, our limits and our possibilities. They help us to feel where we hold back and where we spill out. Our sensuality helps us to be conscious of our being and our becoming.

Sensuality and sexuality are often seen negatively in spiritual circles. They have been exploited within our culture, leaving many people terribly hurt. Our culture is still learning how to honour the sacredness of our bodies, which includes the sensuousness of our senses. As we move to heal our relationship with our sensuality, we can make deeper and safer connections with others. Our sensuality and sexuality are integral parts of feeling alive, and are therefore integral parts of our spirituality.

Not all sexual encounters are deep. Perhaps some people don't want them to be. Like the rest of life, there are ups and downs, times when we feel in sync with others and times we don't. Being with what is, present in and with our bodies as incarnate beings, deeply connected with our sensuality, we meet each other in the present moment and say "Namaste."

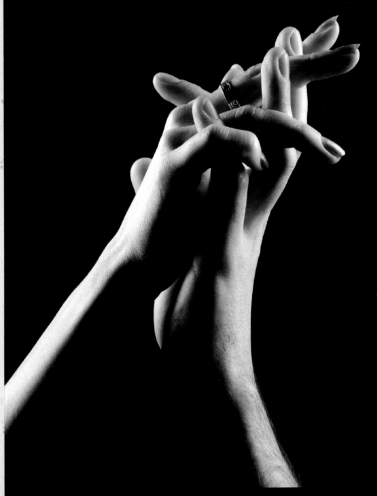

The love on [the heart level of connection] turns your lover into your beloved — and eventually your beloved into the Beloved. This is the level where the mind and body, like you and your beloved, become spiritual collaborators. On this level where bonding occurs, commitment is wholehearted and without interruption. It is here that the romantic notion of the "magic of love" may actually be experienced. When two minds merge in the heart, thought and feelings commingle.

~ Stephen and Ondrea Levine

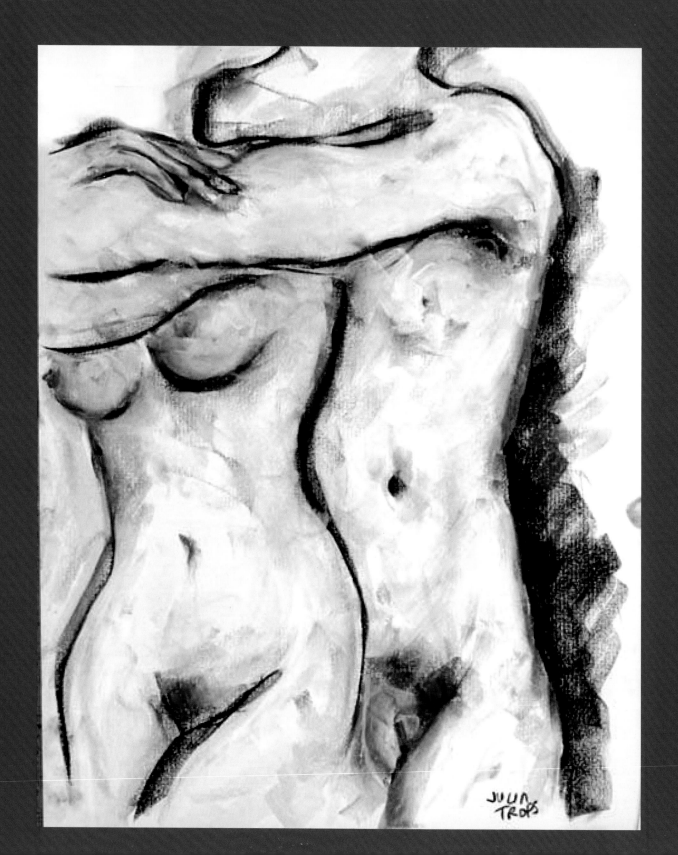

6
Sexual Intimacy

CHARLOTTE JACKSON

If you don't risk anything, you risk even more.

~ ERICA JONG

Oh, curse those fairy tales that promise our redemption through true love and intimacy. The knight on the horse. The princess in the tower. The kiss that brings us to life, that transforms us into the people we always secretly hoped we would become. These stories present a simplistic kind of intimate love that heals all wounds, erases all emptiness, and eradicates all darkness.

True intimate love is both harder than the fairy tale version, and better. It is more challenging, and asks more of us. On the other hand, it is more substantial, more creative, and at the core, transformative.

Don't we all yearn to be transformed, freed, opened up to a greater potential? If we are unable to admit that we yearn for this kind of deliverance, it is likely that we suffer from an acute case of sour grapes! Perhaps we can't admit that we want this kind of relationship because it brings up too many painful feelings of unrequited

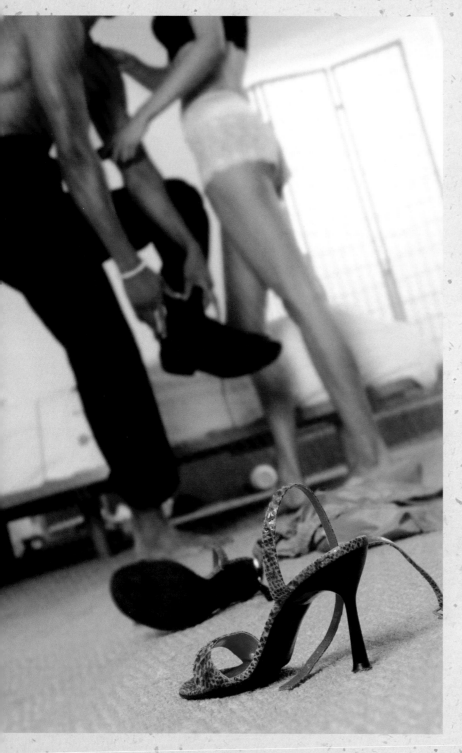

and unfulfilled expectations. We feel it is better to pretend that we never wanted it in the first place and to settle for less, or have nothing at all. Given this state of affairs, how can we begin to look at the issues of intimacy, especially as it pertains to sex, and make any sense of the terrain? If we can't skip to the fairy tale ending, how do we navigate the steps in between?

The nature of sexual intimacy is confusing and complicated. Sexuality comes with significant social baggage, plus a dash of family values mixed in for good measure. On one hand, we are told that sexuality is normal, healthy, human. That it is as natural a force as hunger and thirst. When you are hungry, you eat. When you are thirsty, you drink. And when you feel the stirrings of sexuality? Here begins the complications.

What you believe about your sexuality, your body, and other people affects how your sexuality is expressed. Sexuality and intimacy involve another person, and therefore become a dance of interpersonal dynamics. When it comes to sex, the act is inherently intimate. It involves the closest physical proximity we can achieve with another, second only to being in utero! The relationship, however, may not be intimate at all. The paradox is that a sexual encounter is inherently intimate and yet is so often practiced with casual indifference.

Intimacy 101

Genuinely intimate relationships involve self-knowledge. In order to offer something to another, we need to know what we are giving. This is why sex and marital therapist David Schnarch feels that sexual intimacy is richer as we age. As we mature, we know ourselves better and therefore more poignantly know what we offer – in all our splendour and limitation!

Intimacy is an experience of being close to another – to know a person, to be known by that person, and to genuinely desire to continue moving towards that other with warmth and curiosity and courage. To move towards someone, then, requires that we know what prevents us from moving closer, to know what the barriers are, the obstacles. The issues of trust, honesty, respect, mutuality, eroticism, and love need to be considered. Of course, as we tiptoe through this terrain it is important to maintain a sense of humour. If we take ourselves too seriously we run the risk of digging ourselves into a position and initiating guerrilla warfare rather than nurturing ongoing peace negotiations!

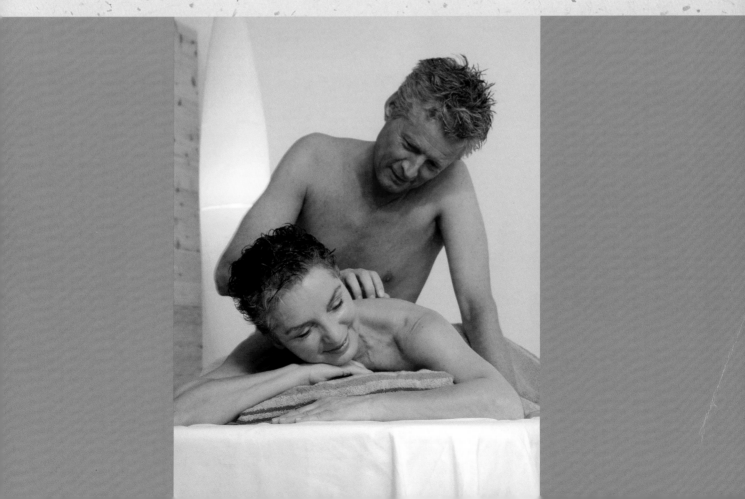

TRUST

To trust another is a leap of faith. To accept the truth of what someone says without evidence is to choose to take the other at face value, to choose to have faith in the other's highest potential. Trust also refers to the state of being responsible for someone else, accountable for another's well-being.

Trust is essential in sexual intimacy. Even couples who practice sexual sadomasochism have a "safety" word, a call for a time out, a signal that "play" is over and limitations need to be respected. This requires significant trust – trust that each partner will be heard and respected.

This goes for intimate relationships of any stripe. In order for sex to be safe, for sexuality to be explored in a rich and dynamic way, both partners must be able to trust in the other, to respect the limits and needs of the other at any given time.

This introduces a para-

dox: in order to risk we need to push boundaries, and yet boundaries are built on trust. We therefore begin to push against issues of trust when we take sexual risks.

Just as trust is built over time, sexual risks need to be taken over time. In order to give the relationship time to grow and adapt, sexual exploration needs to be incremental, organic, reflecting a continuous commitment to the whole of the relationship. To trust, then, is a radical act of optimism; it is to subscribe to a worldview of growth and abundance and potential. It stares scarcity and fear in the face and opts for the bigger, more inclusive stand that we are all connected, interdependent, and guided by a fundamental beneficence.

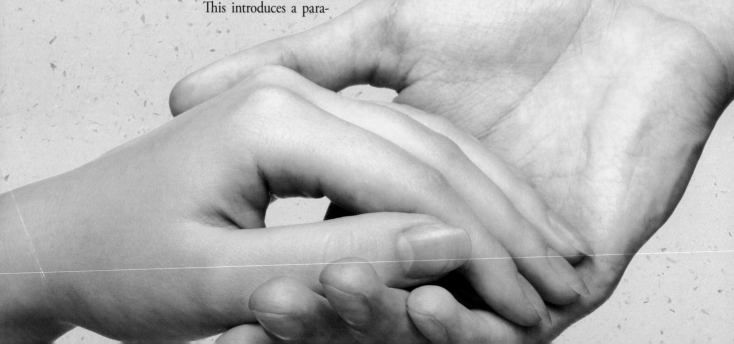

Honesty

To be honest is to conduct one's self with as much sincerity as possible, to strive to be transparent and free of deceit. When we look at the issue of honesty, we must first begin by being honest with ourselves. We can only be as honest with our beloved as we are being honest with ourselves. We need to acknowledge the private stories we nurture about our lover and their shortcomings. This doesn't mean that we share these stories indiscriminately. Unless our lover is asking for feedback, we restrain ourselves from dumping our judgments on them. Mostly we need to take ownership of our judgments and projections and acknowledge how they interfere with being present to who our partner truly is.

We want to leap ahead to the tenderness and sweetness and union of true love. Or we want to remain fixed in the early phases of falling in love. However, in order to fulfill these desires, we must first take an honest look at the part we are playing in our own fairy tale. Often our strategies are the very thing that stand in the way of our realization of the fruits of relationship.

It's a bitter pill to swallow, but the truth is no one else is going to make us happy. No one else is going to rescue us. Like the genie in the bottle waiting to be freed, we sit and wait for the time when someone will come along to emancipate us. We need to change this story. We need to realize that we are the masters of our own fate. As Gandhi said, "*You* must be the change you wish to see in the world."

This is a vulnerable place to be. If we insist on our beloved being the one who needs to change, to be fixed, to somehow be different, we are being dishonest with our own place in the dynamic. The aim of the game is to keep working towards a deeper intimacy. Psychologist George Weinberg said, "Interestingly, the best way to promote intimacy is to demand it." I take this to mean that we must first and foremost demand it of ourselves. We must make intimacy a priority in our own actions rather than waiting for someone else to take charge.

You do not need to wait for the right partner, the right time, the perfect conditions. They may never arrive, or they may already be here. It's only you who arrive, with your aim to deepen your connection in as transparent a manner as possible.

If you choose to stay as you are — and as you are is the very thing holding you back — then it will become far more difficult to experience true intimacy.

- Ian Oshlack

RESPECT

To respect another is to feel a deep admiration for that person, to care about their feelings, wishes, rights, and beliefs. It also refers to a commitment to refrain from harming or interfering with those feelings, wishes, rights, and beliefs. This is a critical ingredient for true sexual intimacy. To respect our beloved is to maintain a fundamental positive regard for them and their sovereignty. As much as we yearn for union and merging in sexual encounters, it must be predicated on a deep respect for our partner's autonomy and self-determination.

Sometimes we rely on manipulation, coercion, or all out bullying to influence our beloved towards meeting our own needs. We often think that things would be simpler, more straightforward, if our partner would just "go along" with us, acquiesce, capitulate. This strategy ultimately backfires. Demand kills desire. We cannot milk love and affection from another through inflicting our will. Intimacy withers under a dictatorship. It is only through a deep commitment to the other's autonomy and difference that we can come together and explore the space between.

There is no shortcut. This requires a capacity to moderate our own need for power and control. This is also an excellent place to practice our sense of humour. We can feel frustrated respecting the otherness of our beloved and moderating our own voracious needs and desires. Lightening up, taking a deep breath, and laughing at our insatiable desires can go a long way to fostering respect for the other.

I think most of the spiritual life is really a matter of relaxing – of what Meister Eckhart called Gelassenheit *– of letting go, ceasing to cling, ceasing to insist on our own way, ceasing to tense ourselves up for this or against that.*
– Beatrice Bruteau

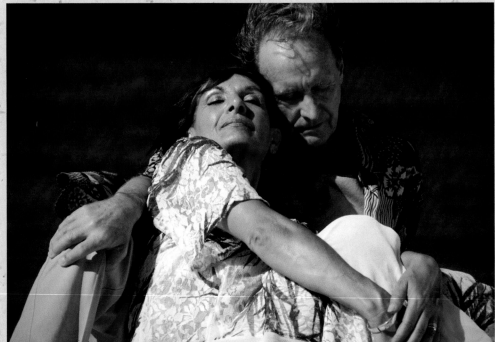

MUTUALITY

Mutuality refers to a commitment to or concern for a common experience, a sense of reciprocity between two people. This has the effect of creating a "field" or condition in which both partners can dwell, a condition of being greater than the sum of the parts.

We are no longer struggling against each other, trying to get our needs met in an environment of diminishing returns. Rather, we are working together towards a deeper and richer intimacy and union.

This is the goal of the left-handed path or tantra. Through the experience of mutu-

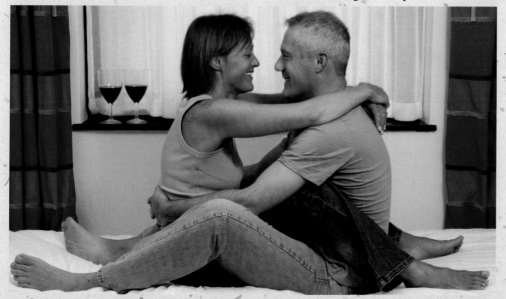

For where two or three are gathered in my name, I am there among them.

~ MATTHEW 18:20

If two lovers devote their energy to their relationship, promote its primacy, they can create a palpable experience of mutuality. Secular life promotes a sense of autonomy, of being separate. We often see life as a series of fractured events: family, work, society, the world at large. We are aware of the divisions, the differences, the separations. What if we shifted our perspective from that of difference and distinction to one of commonality and communion? How would that shift the perspective on our intimate relationships?

ality, of communion with the other, a transcendent state can be achieved. The selfish little me with all its wants and needs is suspended and a greater transformative union emerges. To serve the sexual desires of our beloved, to become a servant to our lover's arousal and ecstasy is to enter into a larger field of generosity and selflessness. In order to do this, we need to make it our job to discover our beloved's sexual barometer, to reveal our own, and to develop and practice together to achieve this higher ground.

EROTICISM

In the expression of sensuality and intimacy, the real thrill is to expect the unexpected.

‑ Ian Oshlack

Eroticism is an essential ingredient in sexual intimacy. While there are naturally times of lassitude in sexual expression, it is the times of charged sexuality that push boundaries, that transform dynamics and deepen connection.

David Schnarch, in his book *Passionate Marriage*, talks about the phenomena of "doing and being done."[1] He devotes a

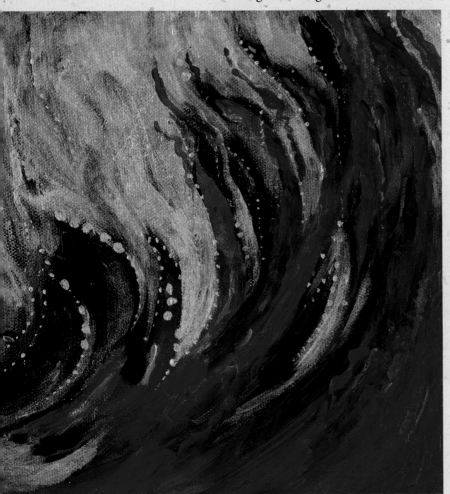

chapter to the experience of the animal side of intimacy. And we do have an animal side. If it is not expressed, it is likely being sublimated and liable to arise somewhere else. Hot sex requires a combination of an open heart and a sense of strength and willpower. Sex that involves an open heart is warm and merging and gentle. It has the qualities of ease and meandering. Sex that involves the genitals alone is largely about power and dominance. This can be exciting, but it is not about love.

Sex that combines the gold of the heart and the red of strength can create conditions for hot sex. Writer David Deida calls it "ravaging."[2] We usually identify ravaging as a destructive act, an activity that wreaks havoc. In the context of hot sex, ravaging does do damage, but to the defences, not the person. It transgresses and transcends the usual barriers and niceties of the personality, penetrating beyond these into uncharted territory.

Drawing this new map can be very helpful to enhancing relationship, not to mention exciting. It can create access to terrain that can only be travelled by lover and beloved together; to a place that cannot be accessed alone.

Of course, there is no erotic formulary. Ravaging, hot sex may be the ideal we hold

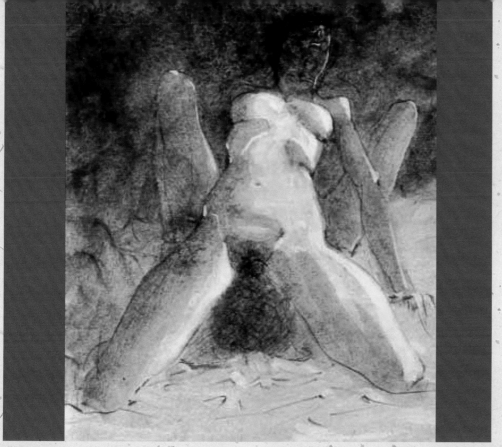

on to when we consider intimate and fulfill-
ing sex. Yet many schools of sexual thought
also stress the importance of ritual and intention, of touch and tentativeness. A light,
tentative touch can be highly arousing.
While ravaging is a fully declared invasion,
a light touch is an invitation, an entice-
ment, a promise that the more you come
out and the more you reveal, the more you
will be met. It is hot and risky. And there is
no hurry, no goal to be achieved.

Meandering in pleasure and arousal can
be a form of meditation, of deep interabiding,
lover in beloved, beloved in lover. We can
learn to surrender to ever-greater pleasure,
to allow it to move beyond the genitals and
permeate throughout the whole body,
opening to the infusion of erotic
pleasure in every cell. This is
vulnerable. And vulner-
ability is at the core
of intimacy.

LOVE

What is love? A strong feeling of affection? A sense of sexual attachment? Or is it truly the only mechanism through which we can intimately know our beloved? It is an act of selfless devotion, a form of voluntary slavery – *voluntary* being the operative word. Feelings, sexual and romantic, come and go. To *really* love someone is, above all, to see them, delight in them, and commit to nurturing their spiritual growth.

This takes effort and courage and time. M. Scott Peck describes love as an intention to support the spiritual growth of another. It is work. It's not just about goodwill and lip service; it's about showing up again and again and again. The position is one of choosing to serve, of being a servant but not a slave – remembering at any given moment that you have a choice to be doing what you are doing, engaging in what you are engaging in.

It is a matter of perspective. Remembering that you always have a choice can alleviate some of the sense of frustration that comes with the struggle for intimacy. When we project on the other our unfulfilled needs, we have to remind ourselves that we choose to be here, creating the dynamic.

The potential in love-based sexuality is a truly transformative union. With deep trust, respect, and honesty, a mutuality can be nurtured from which an ecstatic sexuality can be realized. It is possible to pass from a sense of separation and difference into an experience of enduring bliss and a dance of mutual worship. The safety that comes from developing these conditions creates a portal through which one can pass, from self-consciousness to a sense of timelessness. An intersection between the finite and the infinite. This is a way to acknowledge the divine manifestation in our beloved and in ourselves, and to honour this through all of our senses.

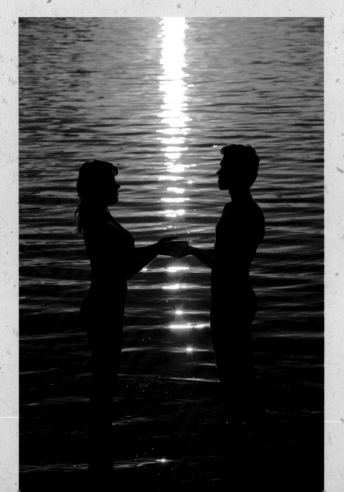

THE ONLY GAME IN TOWN

Love. Sex. Intimacy. All worthy pursuits. What loftier aim, what deeper desire is there than to connect, to be loved, to belong to the human family? But we must realize that we can only manifest love through the other. It is fundamentally an exchange, an outpouring to another and an emptying of ourselves. It is inherently communal. As Hermann Hesse so poignantly said, "If I know what love is, it is because of you."

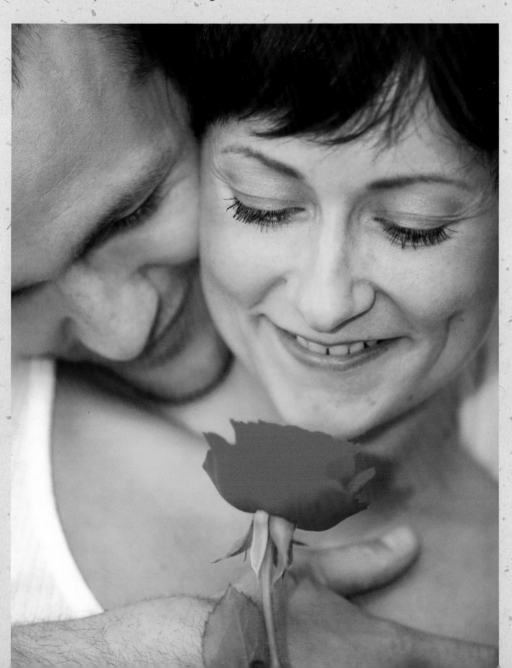

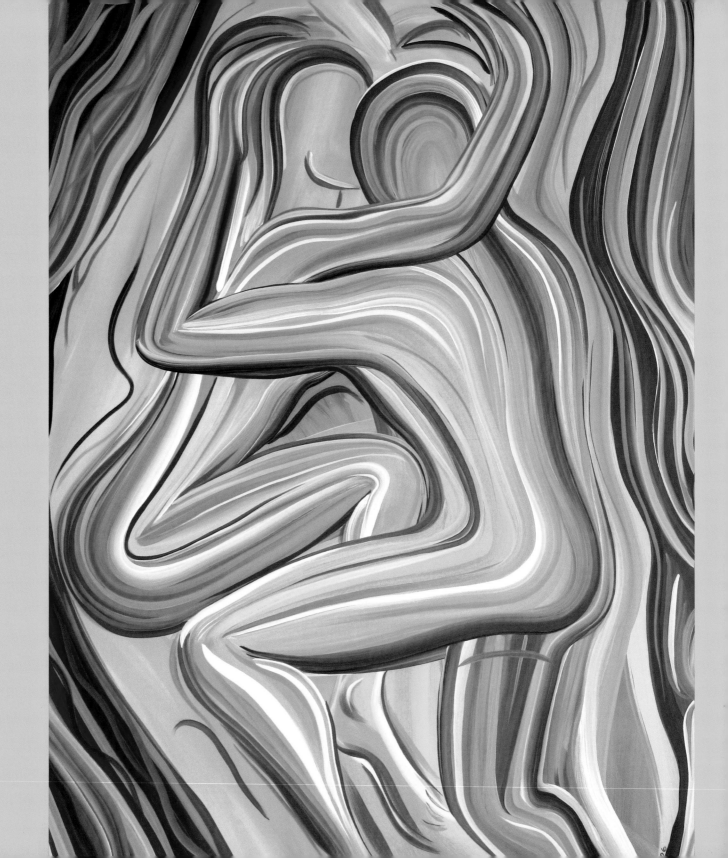

7
The Joy of Sex

MICHAEL SCHWARTZENTRUBER

The erotic... provides the power which comes
from sharing deeply any pursuit with another person.
The sharing of joy, whether physical, emotional, psychic,
or intellectual,
forms a bridge between the sharers...
- AUDRE LORDE

Back in the early 1970s, Alex Comfort wrote a book called *The Joy of Sex*, and for more than 30 years it has remained a popular guide to lovemaking. Like most books of its kind, it focuses on positions and techniques and all the aspects of sex that can enhance a couple's *pleasure*. Nothing wrong with that. Sex *should* be pleasurable, and if it isn't, then something has gone wrong somewhere.

But it's worth pointing out that *pleasure* and *joy* are not exactly the same thing. It is joy, particularly the joy we may discover in sex, that I want to focus on in this final chapter.

Joy is deeper, more profound, more all-encompassing than pleasure. Joy involves the whole self. It suffuses and transforms our entire being. Unlike pleasure, which tends to come from the outside via our

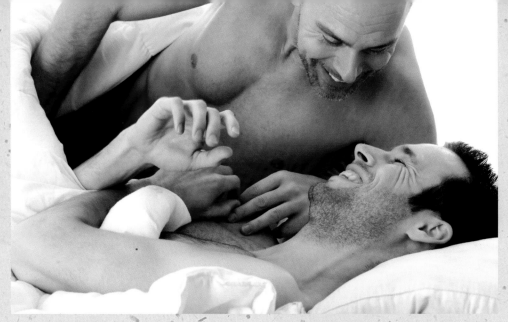

nerve endings and senses and then move inward, joy tends to well up from within and then move outward. We take in or absorb pleasure (we can also give it), but we *radiate* joy.

The joy we experience in sex is no different. Usually it begins on the inside, with the realization that we have discovered a deep, intimate, and loving connection with another human being – a connection that involves a *mutual* knowing of the other. This sense of being known and, at the same time, being accepted and loved fills us with joy. This joy permeates our entire being and affects our *being*, how we are in the world, often so much so that our joy is obvious to others. It radiates from our face, but also perhaps through changed actions and behaviours.

This kind of joy is both spiritual and powerfully erotic in the truest sense. As the Greeks understood it, eros was the magnetism, the force of attraction and desire for union that held the world together. It was also the prime mover that inspired each thing to realize its full potential.

Deep mutual love is capable of all that and more. And so, when we find it, our natural response is joy. One of the most spiritual, intimate, and yes, pleasurable ways we have of expressing and sharing this joy is through sex.

This, then, is the joy of sex. It is the joy that comes from the intimate sharing of the full and true self.

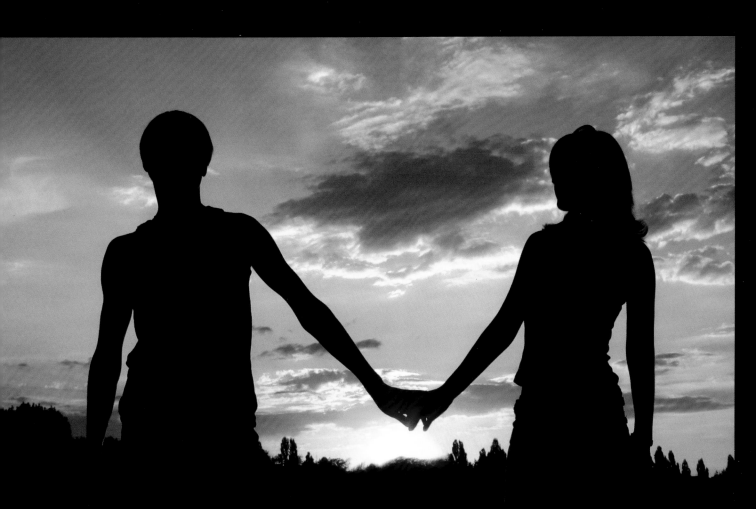

If you were all alone in the universe with no one to talk to, no one with which to share the beauty of the stars, to laugh with, to touch, what would be your purpose in life? It is other life, it is love, which gives your life meaning. This is harmony. We must discover the joy of each other, the joy of challenge, the joy of growth.

~ Mitsugi Saotome

COME PLAY WITH ME AND BE MY LOVE

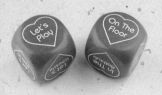

There's another thing about joy that distinguishes it from pleasure. Because of its more complex character, joy tends to be more elusive, a more infrequent visitor to our lives. And while we can usually stimulate our pleasure centres at will and in countless ways, it's often far more difficult to recapture joy once it has flown our lives.

But there is a way, and it's called *play*. Play is the most natural way we have of inviting joy back into our lives. As opposed to competition and games, genuine play, including sex play, is always joyful. It is also highly spiritual.

The idea that play, let alone sexual play, is spiritual does not sit well with everyone. For the most part, play hasn't fared a whole lot better than sex in Western religion. For a great many people for a great portion of history, religion – often the only recognized and sanctioned form of spirituality – has been pretty serious business. It has been freighted with judgment and condemnation and a concern for propriety and proper forms – just like sex.

So to bring the two of them together and suggest that they might be spiritual?

Forget about it!

But it doesn't have to be that way.

Ralph Milton, co-founder of Wood Lake Publishing, likes to say, "Religion is a lot like sex. If you're not having fun, you're not doing it right." When it comes to religion, Ralph is always trying to get people to lighten up, to recognize that God has a sense of humour and fun, maybe even a sense of adventure.

Tom Robbins puts it even more bluntly and colourfully than Ralph, in his novel *Fierce Invalids Home from Hot Climates.*

Suppose the neutral angels were able to talk Yahweh and Lucifer – God and Satan, to use their popular titles – into settling out of court. What would be the terms of the compromise? Specifically, how would they divide the assets of their earthly kingdom?

Would God be satisfied to take loaves and fishes and itty-bitty

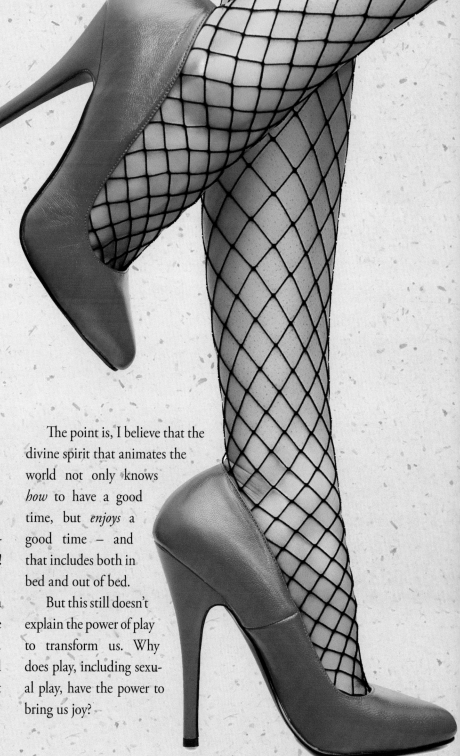

thimbles of Communion wine, while allowing Satan to have the red-eye gravy, eighteen ounce New York steaks, and buckets of chilled champagne? Would God really accept twice-a-month love-making for procreative purposes and give Satan the all-night, no-holds-barred, nasty "can't-get-enough-of-you" hot-as-hell fucks?…

Can anyone see Satan taking pirate radio stations and God being happy with the likes of CBS? God getting twin beds; Satan, water beds…? Would Satan get Harley motorcycles; God, Honda golf carts? Satan get blue jeans and fish-net stockings; God, polyester suits and pantyhose?…

Would almighty God be that dorky? Or would he see rather quickly that Satan was making off with most of the really interesting stuff?[1]

Of course, millions of people would instinctively answer yes to most of those questions! Which may be the problem.

If you ask me, Tom Robbins and Ralph Milton are right. And one look at nature confirms it – God definitely has a wild side. Nature is all about variety and colour and smells and shapes and sounds, much of it very "untamed."

The point is, I believe that the divine spirit that animates the world not only knows *how* to have a good time, but *enjoys* a good time – and that includes both in bed and out of bed.

But this still doesn't explain the power of play to transform us. Why does play, including sexual play, have the power to bring us joy?

Come play with me and be my love and we will some new pleasures prove...
— MICHAEL SCHWARTZENTRUBER, WITH APOLOGIES TO JOHN DONNE (1572–1631)

Sam Keen suggests that it has to do with freeing the spirit, with the freedom we find in play to let go of everything that keeps our true self locked up and fettered: "There is...an innate and nearly indestructible spirit of play in human personality that gives us the capacity to transcend all the molds, morals, masks, and myths that culture would impose on us."[2]

In other words, the experience of joy and the freedom to transcend the strictures imposed by the ego-defined self tend to go hand in hand. It's difficult to experience one without the other. In the quotation below, James Nelson speaks about pleasure, but everything he says applies equally well to the experience of joy.

> To experience the heights of sexual pleasure I must let loose of my need to control. I must let go, giving myself over to the delicious moment. It is a paradox, known in other ways in the gospel but applicable here as well: losing the self means finding the self. Sexual pleasure nurtures the reunion of self with self.[3]

Thomas Moore says pretty much the same thing: "Here is one of the ironies of the soul in sex: deeper pleasure requires an opening to the soul, not just the body, and the soul is full of quirky life. Good sex requires the ability to live from someplace other than the ego."[4]

Joy requires the same thing, and play is one of the best ways to make it happen. Which takes us back to where we started – the intimate and joyful sharing of our unbound selves.

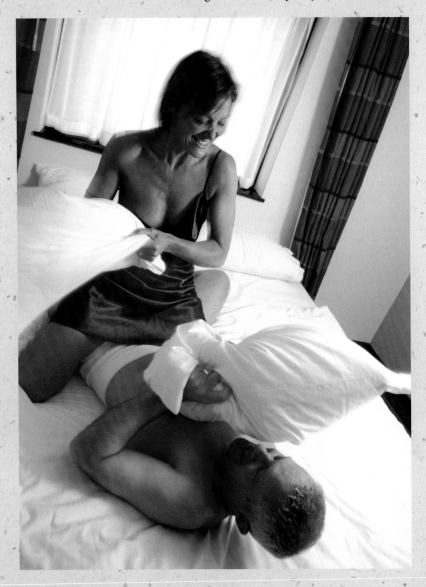

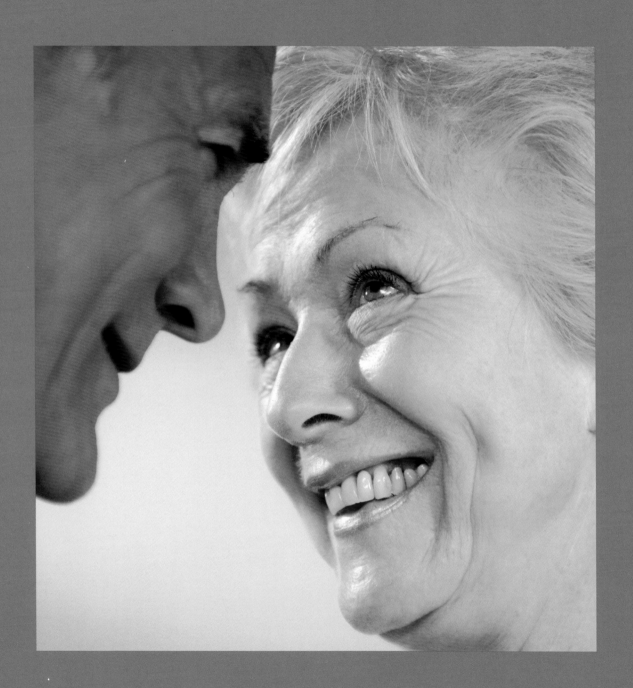

When the Body Betrays, Can It Still Play?

This need to let go of ego, to transcend the small self in order to find joy, is even more critical when our bodies let us down. Or to put it another way, when the body betrays, can it still play?

Susan Ivany, whose husband lives with multiple sclerosis, has had to face this question directly. Here's what she has to say on the subject.

∽

Susan's Perspective

Author Nancy Mairs, like my husband, lives with multiple sclerosis. She has written, among other works, two ground-breaking books on disability and sexual identity: *Remembering the Bone House* and *Carnal Acts*.[5]

Mairs confesses, "I've spent all these years trying alternately to repudiate and to control my wayward body, to transcend it one way or another, but MS rams me right back down into it. Slowly, slowly, MS will teach me how to live on as a body."[6]

In this passage, Mairs is talking about radical acceptance. There is a huge difference between radical acceptance and giving up. Radical acceptance involves surrendering to life's realities and making the best of any given situation. Giving up is an act of despair. It is important to remember that we always have a choice of one or the other.

This is especially important when physical limitations get in the way of perceived norms in sexual activity. Sex and relationships are complicated enough without adding in the hazards of trying to be "normal" – whatever that is. Personal expectations, or those of one's partner, can place a lot of pressure on what should be a pleasurable experience. That pressure itself can inhibit sexual performance.

The good news is that it *is* possible for partners to work together to create new ways of relating to one another sexually while accommodating limits to mobility or movement. In fact, exploring new ways to bring pleasure to your partner can be a great way to nurture your relationship. Of course, not everything you try is going to work. Both partners need to be willing to adapt, explore, talk, and most importantly – laugh. Sex needs to be fun, no matter what your physical abilities.

Thankfully, sex is more than just physical performance. Sex is also relational, mysterious, erotic, exotic, transcendent, and as unique as each human soul.

In a fuller version of the quotation that opens this chapter, Audre Lorde says that

The erotic...provides the power which comes from sharing deeply any pursuit with another person. The sharing of joy, whether physical, emotional, psychic, or intellectual, forms a bridge between the sharers which can be the basis for understanding much of what is not shared between them, and lessens the threat of their difference.[7]

Clearly, we cannot assume anything about *any* person's sexual life. Likewise, we cannot assume to understand the workings of another person's soul simply by looking at them. Matters of the body and the soul are deeply personal and therefore unique.

Our bodies, our spirits, our relationships, our very lives ebb and flow with the circumstances of living. It's not all good. In fact, some of life is just darn awful. Bodies betray. Relationships strain at the challenges of learning a new way to be sexual together.

In all of it, we have the choice to give up and declare life a disaster because it does not compare well to our ideals. But we have another choice as well. We have the option to surrender to life as it *is* instead of waiting for life to become what we would like it to be. We have the option to celebrate life *now*, just as it is, in any way that we are able.

That's called radical acceptance. It may not sound very sexy, but trust me, it is.

၏

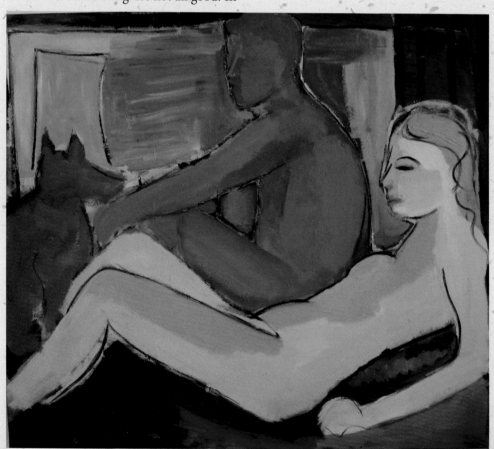

TRANSFORMATIONAL SEX

When it comes to sex and spirituality, the kind of radical self-acceptance and the ability to surrender to what *is* that Susan describes – the ability to let go of our need to control, and give ourselves over to the moment, to paraphrase Nelson – is precisely what can lift us, regardless of our physical abilities, above and beyond the bounds of ordinary experience.

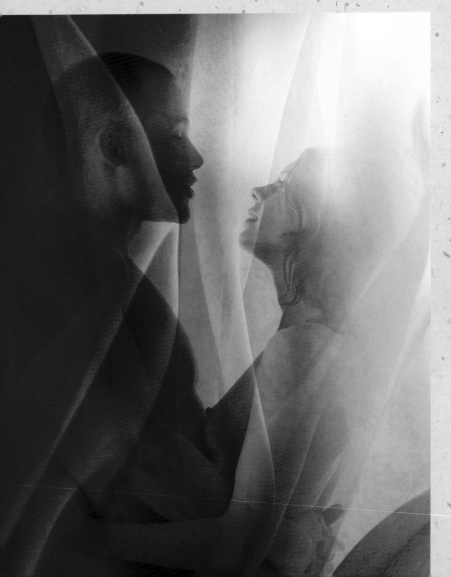

There are lots of names for this kind of transcendent sexual-spiritual experience. Some call it sacred sex, others mystical sex, and still others call it oceanic sex. David Schnarch, a sex and marital therapist, learned the term "wall socket sex" from his clients. The term, he says, refers to the "sustained electric jolt of sex on the boundaries." Wall socket sex, he continues,

involves physical and emotional union in the context of consuming mutual desire, heart-stopping intimacy, and deep meaningfulness. It includes multiple levels of psychological involvement and taps all capacities that are uniquely human, including mutuality, integrity, and spirituality.[8]

Clearly, this is about much more than a good orgasm or even multiple orgasms. In fact, it's not about orgasms at all, although they may certainly play a role in the experience. It's about emotional, physical, and spiritual connection on a deeply interior and yet paradoxically transcendent level, as can be seen from the kinds of experiences people report:

- Time stops.
- External reality fades; there may be a sense of being transported to another time and place.

- Separate acts blend into a single moment or event.
- Boundaries – emotional, physical, or spiritual – between partners shift or cease to exist. You *feel* your partner without touching.
- Your emotions appear on your partner's face.
- You watch your partner undergo age changes. You know exactly what he or she looked like in childhood, or will look like when older.
- Profound mutual caring and joy overflow the bond between you.[9]

Often, the feeling of connection people describe includes a sense of deep union with God, Goddess, the Divine, a Higher Power – the words people use to name the holy are many – and with the Earth and all that *is*. This *unio mystica* or mystical union with the Divine is typically accompanied by an experience of spiritual ecstasy, a form of joy known particularly well by the ancient love mystics.

But perhaps the most important part of these experiences, the reason they are spiritual in the deepest sense, is the power they have to bring about positive, creative growth and change.

One woman I know described exactly this kind of experience and the transformative power it had on her.

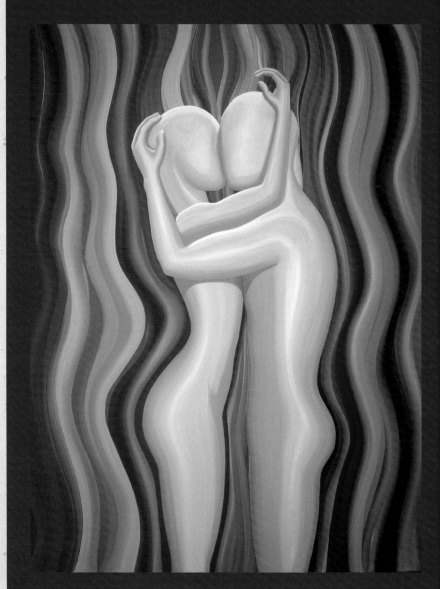

I tell you, deep inside you is a fountain of bliss, a fountain of joy. Deep inside your center core is truth, light, love. There is no guilt there, there is no fear there. Psychologists have never looked deep enough.

~ Ravi Shankar

It was an amazing time with my new partner – making love was not just a physical experience, but for me, spiritual and transformational as well.

My partner took the time to light candles to set the mood. Awakening all the senses was an important part of our love-making – soft music, scented and sensuous oils, gentle caresses, the sound of our breathing, the taste of skin. As we looked into each other's eyes there was love. Our bodies became an extension of that love. We felt free to be ourselves without inhibition or judgment. The amazing thing is that it felt so right and sacred to show our love for each other with our whole self – our body, mind, and soul.

Our bodies, the room, the world were infused with deep joy and thanksgiving that spilled over into the rest of the hours of the day. I became more creative, more open, more caring. This was the exact opposite of a previous relationship where criticism and lack of respect had shriveled my heart and soul. Now it was like the sun had come out bringing warmth and life-giving energy. In this new relationship it felt like I could once again grow and come to life.

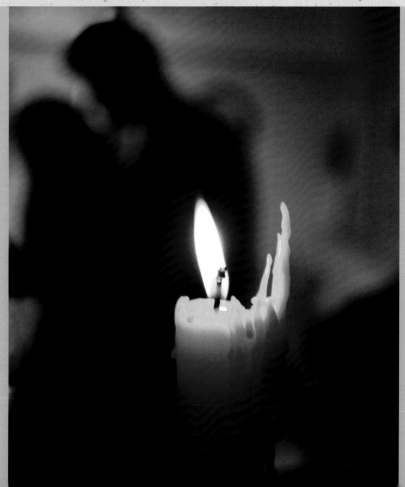

It has often been said that when it comes to sex, the most important organ is the not the genitals, but the brain. To be honest, I'm not sure there *is* a most important part or organ. And if I *were* making a list to choose from, I would include more than just the genitals and the brain, the body and the mind. I would also want to include the heart and the soul.

The truth is that sex at its full spiritual potential involves all of these mixed together to form a complex and powerful elixir that has the power to transform our lives. Which is why I like this woman's story so much. Her experience encapsulates perfectly so many of the things we have tried to say in this book.

Sex at its full spiritual potential is about embracing the body and all the gifts it has to offer. But it is also about so much more than just the body. It is about relationships and love, trust and integrity, respect and awareness, beauty and passion, play and pleasure, thankfulness and joy. It is about freedom and safety, acceptance and encouragement, creativity and change, transformation and fulfillment. It is about birth and death, living and dying, rising and falling, ending and starting over.

In short, it is about everything that makes us human and humane. And that is cause for celebration and joy indeed.

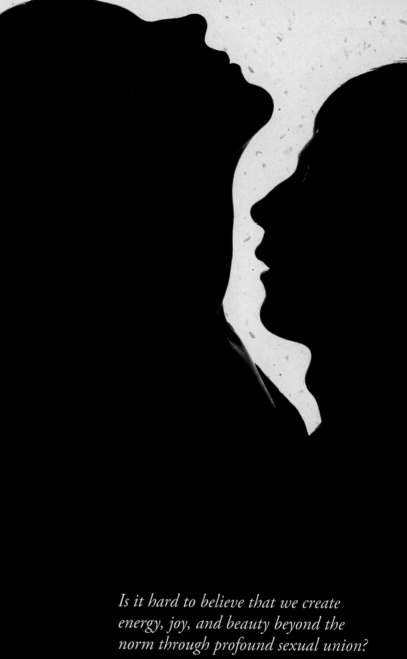

Is it hard to believe that we create energy, joy, and beauty beyond the norm through profound sexual union?

- DAVID SCHNARCH

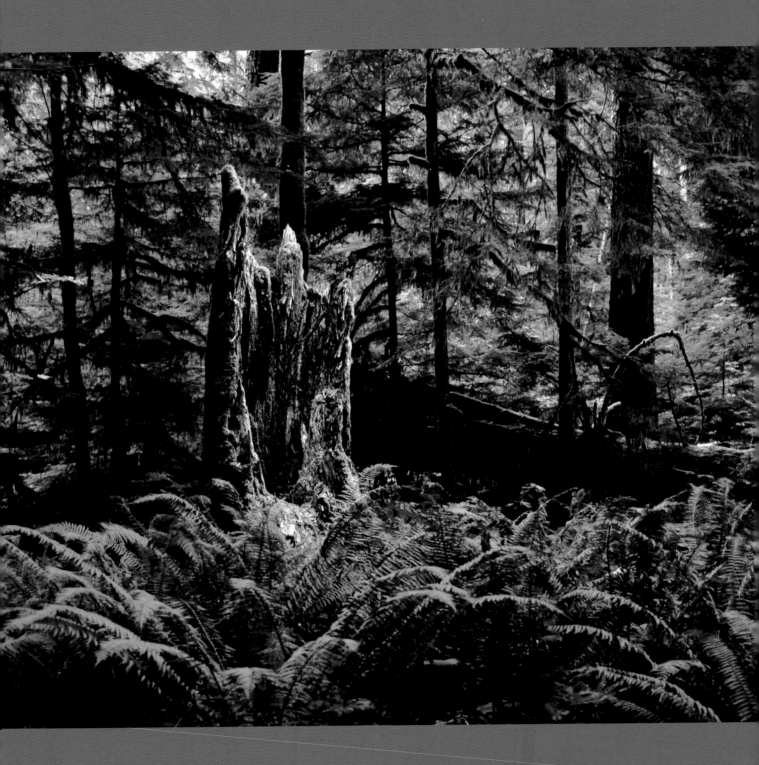

Ecology and the Erotic Spirit

MICHAEL SCHWARTZENTRUBER

*At the deepest level,
knowledge is the awareness of our participation in the
reality of the other.
Ignorance is based on the illusion of our separation.*
~ SAM KEEN

No doubt some people will have looked at this book and thought, "Not another book on sex! Don't these people know what's happening in the world? Don't they have anything better to do with their time?" And to be honest, during the year and a half of writing, we have sometimes been four of those people.

This planet and the vast multitude of life forms that inhabit it are not in great shape. Nor is the situation getting better.

Temperatures are rising, food crops are failing, the ice caps are melting, sea levels are rising, fresh water is disappearing. And in far too many places, people are dying from hunger and thirst and malnutrition, or from preventable diseases, or from war or other forms of violence, or from any number of other things that are the direct result of social and economic injustice.

Meanwhile, the plant and animal kingdoms are suffering equally great threats. We

The prevailing view has been that the body… is a fragment of the Universe, a piece completely detached from the rest and handed over to the spirit that informs it. In the future we shall have to say that the Body is the very Universality of things… My matter is not a part of the Universe that I possess totaliter: *it is the totality of the Universe possessed by me* partialiter.

— Teilhard de Chardin

are, in fact, living through what scientists now call the "sixth great extinction," as untold numbers of species disappear forever – fish, fowl, amphibians, mammals, and plant life alike.

We have been very much aware of all of this as we have worked on this book, and we have sometimes wondered why we would bother to continue.

But time after time we were drawn forward by the erotic vision and wisdom of the scholars and sages we were reading – a vision and wisdom confirmed by evolution and the emerging sciences.

Climate change, extinction, food and water shortages, disease, war, and other forms of social unrest – all of them will thrive so long as we continue to live under the "illusion of our separation." All of them will thrive so long as we continue to

understand ourselves, other species, and the planet itself as disconnected, each from the other.

But gone are the days when we can afford to perpetuate the myth of our separateness – one human tribe from another, human life from the lives of other-than-human species, and the lives of all living things from the well-being of the planet as a whole. Gone are the days when we can afford to perpetuate the myth that we somehow stand alone and apart from everything else that is, or that we can somehow escape the consequences of our actions. What befalls creation befalls us.

While there are no easy solutions to the challenges we face, scientists and sages alike have declared loudly and with one voice the truth of our existence. We live and move and have our being within a web of *being*

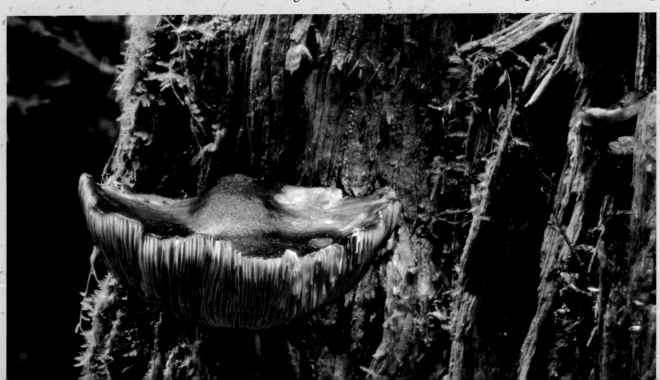

that is interconnected, interrelated, and interdependent in all its aspects.

This being so, the best hope we have of healing the planet, the environment, and even the deep rifts that divide the human family, lies in our ability and willingness to recover a truly erotic sensibility. Eros is all about the connection between beings and the *desire* for that connection. Today, perhaps, we should say it is all about the desire for *re*-connection, for *re*-union.

In this sense, the desire many of us feel to spend time in nature is an *erotic* desire, and the awe and spiritual connection we experience when we open our eyes to the beauty we find there is deeply erotic as well. In other words, the erotic energy we manifest in our lovemaking is only one expression of a larger erotic force that has the power to bind and heal the wounds of the world.

How can we help this healing happen? In this, as with many things, it is okay to begin small. We can begin by recognizing the sacred in the most ordinary circumstances and activities: preparing food and taking the time to enjoy it; playing with our children; tending our gardens; and yes, making love.

In short, we need to recover our erotic vision, develop an understanding of that vision as sacred, and extend it into all aspects of our living. If this book has helped you take even a small step towards this goal, then we are well pleased.

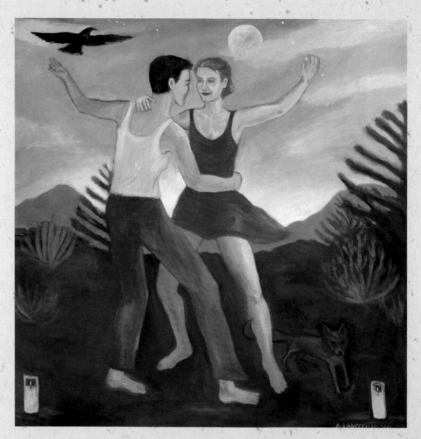

Sexual love is both most passionate and most ordered when it assumes its rightful position within a nexus of erotic relationships that make up the natural world. Earthly love begins when we acknowledge our participation in an ecological bonding that joins all the species of life in a single commonwealth.

~ SAM KEEN

155

ENDNOTES

Chapter 1

1 Thomas Moore, *The Soul of Sex: Cultivating Life as an Act of Love* (New York: HarperPerennial, 1998), 3.

2 As quoted in Matthew Fox, *One River, Many Wells: Wisdom Springing from Global Faiths* (New York: Jeremy P. Tarcher/Putnam, 2000), 310.

3 Hafiz, *The Subject Tonight Is Love: 60 Wild and Sweet Poems of Hafiz*, trans. Daniel Ladinsky (New York: Penguin Compass, 2003), 45.

4 Sam Keen, *The Passionate Life: Stages of Loving* (New York: Harper & Row, 1983), 15–17.

5 Ibid., 17–18.

6 Ibid., 18.

7 Ibid., 25.

8 Matthew Fox, *Sins of the Spirit, Blessings of the Flesh: Lessons for Transforming Evil in Soul and Society* (New York: Three Rivers Press, 1999), 211.

9 As quoted in Moore, *Soul of Sex*, 33.

10 Ibid., 34.

11 Robert Bly and Marion Woodman, *The Maiden King: The Reunion of Masculine and Feminine* (New York: Henry Holt and Company, 1998), 22.

Chapter 2

1 Georg Feuerstein, *Sacred Sexuality: The Erotic Spirit in the World's Great Religions* (Rochester, VT: Inner Traditions, 2003), 53–54.

2 Diane Wolkstein and Samuel N. Kramer, *Inanna: Queen of Heaven and Earth* (New York: Harper & Row, 1983) as quoted in Feuerstein, *Sacred Sexuality*, 58.

3 Ibid., 59.

4 Ibid., 62. See also "Watching as Life Begins: the Discovery of the Mammalian Ovum and the Process of Fertilization" from *Science and Its Times*. © 2005-2006 Thomson Gale, a part of the Thomson Corporation. http://www.bookrags.com/research/watching-as-life-begins-the-discove-scit-0512

5 Moore, *Soul of Sex*, 41, 42.

6 Teresa J. Hornsby, *Sex Texts from the Bible: Selections Annotated & Explained* (Woodstock, VT: SkyLight Paths Publishing, 2007), 171.

7 Feuerstein, *Sacred Sexuality*, 96.

8 As quoted in an article by W. Jay Wood, "What Would Augustine Say? Sex: God's Blessing or Humanity's Curse," Christianity Today Library.com, July 1, 2000. http://www.ctlibrary.com/ch/2000/issue67/10.36.html In later years, Augustine softened his stance and acknowledged that sex for procreation within marriage might actually be okay, but he remained personally committed to the ideal of sexual abstinence.

9 To its credit, the Roman Catholic Church declared marriage a sacrament in the 12th century forming the basis for a positive view of sexual love within marriage that was a break with Augustine. In the 1500s, the Protestant Reformers took this a step further and affirmed the goodness and sacredness of marriage and marital sex for everyone, including clergy.

10 As quoted in Monica Furlong, *Visions and Longings: Medieval Women Mystics* (Boston: Shambhala, 1996), 114.

11 As quoted in Tessa Bielecki, *Teresa of Avila: Ecstasy and Common Sense* (Boston: Shambhala, 1996), 106.

12 Ibid., 110.

13 As quoted in Matthew Fox, *One River, Many Wells*, 314.

14 Ibid.

15 For information on the male and female aspects of the divine and their union, see the article at http://en.wikipedia.org/wiki/Zohar and the references to *Eros and Kabbalah*, by Moshe Idel.

16 Feuerstein, *Sacred Sexuality*, 122.

17 From *The Gift: Poems by Hafiz the Great Sufi Master*, trans. Daniel Ladinsky (New York: Penguin Compass, 1999), 140.

18 From *The Essential Rumi*, trans. Coleman Barks with John Moyne (Edison, NJ: Castle Books, 1997), 135–136.

19 Feuerstein, *Sacred Sexuality*, 135.

20 L. A. Narain, *Khajuraho: Ecstasy in Indian Sculpture* (New Delhi: Roli Books International, 1982), 37.

21 Ibid., 205.

Chapter 3

1 Marion Woodman, *The Pregnant Virgin: A Process of Psychological Transformation* (Toronto: Inner City Books, 1985), 153.

2 Marion Woodman, *Emily Dickinson and The Demon Lover*, Audiobook (Boulder: Sounds True Recordings, 1993).

3 John A. Sanford, *The Invisible Partners: How the Male and Female in Each of Us Affects Our Relationships* (New York: Paulist Press, 1980), 118.

4 Alice Walker, *The Color Purple* (New York: Harcourt Brace Jovanovich, 1982), 192.

5 Ibid., 196.

6 Mary D. Pellauer, "The Moral Significance of Female Orgasm: Toward Sexual Ethics that Celebrates Women's Sexuality," James Nelson and Sandra Longfellow, eds., *Sexuality and the Sacred: Sources for Theological Reflection* (Louisville, KY: Westminster John Knox, 1994), 149–168.

Chapter 4

1 Sarah Hampson, "Sex, or he's your ex," in *The Globe and Mail* (June 7, 2007).

2 Bernie Zilbergeld, *The New Male Sexuality: The Truth about Men, Sex, and Pleasure* (New York: Bantam, 1999), 15–34.

3 James B. Nelson, *The Intimate Connection: Male Sexuality, Masculine Spirituality* (Philadelphia: The Westminster Press, 1988), 14.

4 Zilbergeld, *New Male Sexuality*, 107.

5 Nelson, *Intimate Connection*, 22.

6 Ibid., 23.

7 Ibid., 95.

8 Ibid., 96.

Chapter 5

1 Eugene T. Gendlin, *Focusing* (New York: Bantam Books, 1981), 33.

2 Thomas Keating, *Open Mind Open Heart: The Contemplative Dimension of the Gospel* (New York: Continuum, 1992) 34–35.

3 Bernard McGinn, *The Flowering of Mysticism: Men and Women in the New Mysticism – 1200–1350* (New York: The Crossroad Publishing Company, 1998), 172.

4 Ibid., 218.

5 Daniel Siegel M.D., *The Neurobiology of We: How Relationships, the Mind and the Brain Interact to Shape Who We Are* (Boulder: Sounds True Audio Learning Course).

6 David Schnarch, *Passionate Marriage: Keeping Love and Intimacy Alive in Committed Relationships* (New York: Owl Books, Henry Holt and Company, 1998), 157–186.

7 John R. Haule, *The Love Cure: Therapy Erotic and Sexual* (Connecticut: Spring Publishing, Inc., 1996), 32.

Chapter 6

1 Schnarch, *Passionate Marriage*, 261–287.

2 David Deida, *The Way of the Superior Man: A Spiritual Guide to Mastering the Challenges of Women, Work, and Sexual Desire* (Louisville, CO: Sounds True, 2004).

Chapter 7

1 Tom Robbins, *Fierce Invalids Home from Hot Climates* (New York: Bantam Books, 2000), 287.

2 Keen, *The Passionate Life*, 45.

3 Nelson, *The Intimate Connection*, 59.

4 Moore, *Soul of Sex*, 235.

5 Nancy Mairs, *Remembering the Bone House: An Erotics of Place and Space* (New York: Harper & Row, Publishers, 1989) and *Carnal Acts* (New York: HarperCollins, 1990).

6 As quoted in Nancy L. Eiesland, *The Disabled God: Toward a Liberatory Theology of Disability* (Nashville: Abingdon Press, 1994), 43.

7 Ibid., 96.

8 Schnarch, *Passionate Marriage*, 96.

9 Adapted from Schnarch, *Passionate Marriage*, 97.

BIBLIOGRAPHY AND RECOMMENDED READING

Barks, Coleman, trans. *The Essential Rumi.* with John Moyne. Edison, NJ: Castle Books, 1997.

Bielecki, Tessa. *Teresa of Avila: Ecstasy and Common Sense.* Boston: Shambhala, 1996.

Bly, Robert and Marion Woodman. *The Maiden King: The Reunion of Masculine and Feminine.* New York: Henry Holt and Company, 1998.

Camphausen, Rufus C. *Encyclopedia of Erotic Wisdom: A Reference Guide to the Symbolism, Techniques, Rituals, Sacred Texts, Psychology, Anatomy and History of Sexuality.* Rochester, VT: Inner Traditions International, 1991.

Cattrall, Kim. *Sexual Intelligence.* Vancouver: Greystone, 2005.

Deida, David. *The Way of the Superior Man: A Spiritual Guide to Mastering the Challenges of Women, Work, and Sexual Desire.* Louisville, CO: Sounds True, 2004.

Feuerstein, Georg. *Sacred Sexuality: The Erotic Spirit in the World's Great Religions.* Rochester, VT: Inner Traditions, 2003.

Fox, Matthew. *One River, Many Wells: Wisdom Springing from Global Faiths.* New York: Jeremy P. Tarcher/Putnam, 2000.

— *Sins of the Spirit, Blessings of the Flesh: Lessons in Transforming Evil in Soul and Society.* New York: Three Rivers Press, 1999.

Furlong, Monica. *Visions and Longings: Medieval Women Mystics.* Boston: Shambhala, 1996.

Gendlin, Eugene T. *Focusing.* New York: Bantam Books, 1981.

Haule, John R. *The Love Cure: Therapy Erotic and Sexual.* Connecticut: Spring Publishing, Inc., 1996.

Hickling, Meg. *Meg Hickling's Grown-up Sex: Sexual Wholeness for the Better Part of your Life.* Kelowna, BC: Northstone, 2008.

Hornsby, Teresa J. *Sex Texts from the Bible: Selections Annotated & Explained.* Woodstock, VT: Skylight Paths Publishing, 2007.

Johnson, Robert A. *We: Understanding the Psychology of Romantic Love.* New York: Harper & Row, 1983. (See also the books *She, He,* and *Ecstasy* all by the same author and publisher.)

Keating, Thomas. *Open Mind Open Heart: The Contemplative Dimension of the Gospel.* New York: Continuum, 1992.

Keen, Sam. *The Passionate Life: Stages of Loving.* San Francisco: Harper & Row Publishers, 1983.

Ladinsky, Daniel, trans. *The Gift: Poems by Hafiz the Great Sufi Master.* New York: Penguin Compass, 1999.

— *The Subject Tonight Is Love: 60 Wild and Sweet Poems of Hafiz.* New York: Penguin Compass, 2003.

McGinn. Bernard. *The Flowering of Mysticism: Men and Women in the New Mysticism – 1200-1350.* New York: The Crossroad Publishing Company, 1998.

Moore, Thomas. *The Soul of Sex: Cultivating Life as an Act of Love.* New York: HarperPerennial, 1998.

Mueller-Nelson, Gertrude. *Here All Dwell Free: Stories to Heal the Wounded Feminine.* New York: Doubleday, 1991.

Narain, L. A. *Khajuraho: Ecstasy in Indian Sculpture.* New Delhi: Roli Books, 1982.

Nelson, James B. *The Intimate Connection: Male Sexuality, Masculine Spirituality.* Philadelphia: The Westminster Press, 1988.

Nelson, James B. and Sandra P. Longfellow, eds. *Sexuality and the Sacred: Sources for Theological Reflection.* Louisville, KY: Westminster John Knox Press, 1994.

Salmonsohn, Karen. *The Clitourist: A Guide to One of the Hottest Spots on Earth.* Illustrated by Trisha Krauss. New York: Universe Publishing, 2001.

Sanford, John A. *The Invisible Partners: How the Male and Female in Each of Us Affects Our Relationships.* New York: Paulist Press, 1980.

Schnarch, David. *Passionate Marriage: Keeping Love & Intimacy Alive in Committed Relationships.* New York: Henry Holt. 1998.

Siegel, Daniel, M.D. *The Neurobiology of We: How Relationships, the Mind and the Brain Interact to Shape Who We Are.* Boulder, CO: Sounds True Audio Learning Course.

Tannahill, Reay. *Sex in History.* Briarcliff Manor, NY: Scarborough House/Publishers, 1992.

Walker, Barbara G. *The Woman's Encyclopedia of Myths and Secrets.* New York: Harper & Row, 1983.

— *The Woman's Dictionary of Symbols and Sacred Objects.* New York: Harper & Row, 1990.

Woodman, Marion. *The Pregnant Virgin.* Toronto: Inner City Books, 1985.

Zilbergeld, Bernie. *The New Male Sexuality: The Truth about Men, Sex, and Pleasure.* New York: Bantam, 1999.

CREDITS

All photos and artwork is used by permission.

159

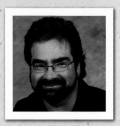 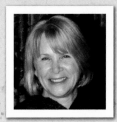 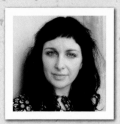 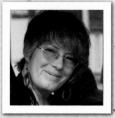

MICHAEL SCHWARTZENTRUBER is associate publisher for Wood Lake Publishing and was for many years the editorial director for its Woodlake, Northstone, and CopperHouse imprints. He has spent much of his life reflecting on the role of sex and sexuality in the spiritual life, and has edited several books on sexual health and childhood sexual health education. He lives in Okanagan Centre, British Columbia, with his wife, Margaret.

MARY MILLERD, MATS (Master of Arts in Theological Studies), is a spiritual director and teacher. She teaches spiritual formation and energy awareness classes for individuals, couples, and groups. She has a certificate in Family Systems Therapy as well as a certificate in Bodynamics Shock Trauma Training Program. Mary integrates her understanding of Somatic Psychotherapy and Family Systems Therapy into her teaching and her spiritual direction sessions.

CHARLOTTE JACKSON is a Registered Clinical Counsellor working in Vancouver, British Columbia. She divides her time between Vancouver's Downtown Eastside, where she is a trauma counselor, and her private practice where she works with couples and individuals addressing relationship issues. Charlotte has been interested in the topic of sexuality for many years, especially as it pertains to intimacy, self-expression, and its intersection with the spiritual realm. She has studied with Father Thomas Keating and is an ongoing student of the Ridhwan School.

LOIS HUEY-HECK is a spiritual director, retreat leader/group facilitator, author and visual artist. For over twenty years her day job (spiritual publishing) also connected her to matters of spirituality and the practical concerns of putting values/beliefs into action. She has an abiding belief in the inherent sacredness of the body and all creation. The symbiotic relationship between sexuality and spirituality remains a favourite subject in her art, writing and research.

THE *Spirituality* OF...

These beautiful books make excellent gifts!

This ever-popular series is ten titles strong!

Other titles in this series are:

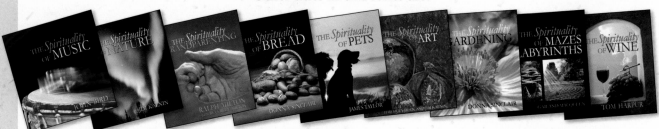

The Spirituality of Music
by John Bird

The Spirituality of Nature
by Jim Kalnin

The Spirituality of Grandparenting
by Ralph Milton with Beverley Milton

The Spirituality of Bread
by Donna Sinclair

The Spirituality of Pets
by James Taylor

The Spirituality of Art
by Lois Huey-Heck and Jim Kalnin

The Spirituality of Gardening
by Donna Sinclair

The Spirituality of Mazes & Labyrinths
by Gailand MacQueen

The Spirituality of Wine
by Tom Harpur

Available at fine bookstores or online at www.woodlakebooks.com or call 1.888.841.9991